Kitchenary

Kitchenary

Birth to Zucchini

A Memoir

Peggy H. Landis

Copyright © 2013 by Kitchenary.

Cover photographs by Jon Styer

Library of Congress Control Number: 2013901303
ISBN: Hardcover 978-1-4797-8351-9
       Softcover 978-1-4797-8350-2
       Ebook   978-1-4797-8352-6

All rights reserved. No part of this book may be reproduced or transmitted in any form or by any means, electronic or mechanical, including photocopying, recording, or by any information storage and retrieval system, without permission in writing from the copyright owner.

This book was printed in the United States of America.

To order additional copies of this book, contact:
Xlibris Corporation
1-888-795-4274
www.Xlibris.com
Orders@Xlibris.com
124930

Contents

A

Aging 15
Antiquing 18

B

Books And Reading 23

C

Chicago Avenue 31
Christmas 34
Coventry Cathedral 40

D

Daddy 45
Declensions And Conjugations 49

E

England 55

F

Farm Food 65
Foreign Hospitality 70
Fountain 83

G

Grandchilden 89
Grandparents Heatwole 96
Grandparents Suter 104

H

Home 115

I

Idaho: Part One 123
Idaho: Part Two 129

J

Jim 139
Journaling 142
Julian Of Norwich 144

K

Keezletown Childhood 149

L

Landis And Good Families 157

M

Mother: Her Later Years 165

N

Neighborhood With A View 173

O

Ornamental Tour 179
Ouch And Ounce 184

P

Park View Mennonite Church 191
Photographs 197

Q

Quilt Story 207

R

Roses 215

S

Sisters, Seekers, Small Group 223
Student 230

T

Thimble Collection 237
Twins! 242

U

Uncles, Aunts, And Cousins 253

V

Volunteer 261

W

Work Wrap-Up 269

XYZ

Xyz: A Conclusion 281

to

Mother
for
her nurture and nutrition

and to

Jay
who is my centerpiece

The "best" preparation is the one that transports people elsewhere, far away from the table.

—Jaspreet Singh, *Chef,* Bloomsbury, 2010

Preface

From birth to the unknown—why did I write this memoir? My answer is that my great-grandmother did not write her story. I know so little about Mary Heatwole Showalter (1862-1950) who was already seventy-seven when I was born. What were her thoughts as she tilted back and forth, back and forth, in her rocking chair, remembering the past, reaching for the new beginning? If she could have written those thoughts and stories, I could read them.

Now I am the fulcrum in a six-generation span, the only one who glimpsed my grandchildren's great-great-great-grandmother. My mother said Great-Grandmother made the best chicken and noodles Mother ever ate, one of the few extant testimonials to her legacy. Yet how important that fact is because it reinforces my knowledge that the sight, smell, and taste of particular foods evoke memories of particular people, places, and incidents. Food, our universal need and pleasure, spans the generations.

I have Great-Grandmother's sparkling cut-glass compote with fluted rim and ornate stem. I imagine her satisfaction as she filled it with fruit and placed it in the center of her dining room table before her guests arrived.

This story is for you, my great-granddaughters and sons, whenever you may be, and it is for anyone who wonders about the life of an average churchgoing woman living and working in the Shenandoah Valley of Virginia when the calendar page of a new millennium was turned.

I set the compote on my table and invite you to read my story.

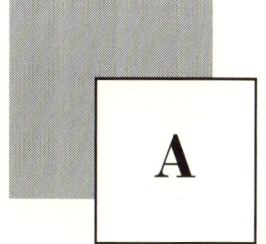

\'ā\ (also a)
n. (pl. as or a's)
the first letter of the alphabet

AGING

Recipe: Fresh Fruit with Orange Glaze

ANTIQUING

Recipe: Ham Pot Pie

AGING

The sun at noon is the sun declining;
The person born is the person dying.

—Unknown

I was born at home in an old Rockingham County farmhouse. President Franklin D. Roosevelt, in his White House worrying about the rumbles of impending World War II, took no notice. Nor did Eleanor. However, the blossoms in the neighboring Oceola Orchard had formed into fruit and waited to be harvested.

When I gave notice of my approaching delivery, the expectant father summoned a kind neighbor, Mrs. Pearl Minnick, to stay with my mother while he drove off in the unreliable Ford coupe to bring the doctor. Some hours went by.

I was the firstborn, and my mother had no prior knowledge of the stages of labor. What had happened to her husband? When would the doctor arrive? At long last, he and the doctor returned and told the story of how one of the back wheels of the coupe had spun off the car and had to be remounted.

Actually, there was no hurry. I knew it was time, but I hesitated to leave my safe place. Maybe I too heard the distant rumbles of war in the world out there. M. S. Foster, MD, of Bridgewater, Virginia, began to lay out the tools for a delivery with forceps. The threat of such violence moved me to action; and soon I emerged, a seven-pound baby girl, somewhat birth marked by the traumatic experience but ready to breathe on my own.

It was Monday, August 7, 1939.

My birth certificate states that I was the full-term legitimate white child of Roy Abram Heatwole, twenty-four, who was employed at the silk mill, and Dorothy Frances Suter, twenty-one, who was a housekeeper in her own home at Mount Crawford, Virginia.

Many birthdays passed. In 2009, I turned seventy.

Two friends, Miriam Martin and Ann Yoder, and I discovered that we all would be turning seventy within six weeks of each other. Thrilled by our parallel pilgrimages, we determined to throw a grand celebration for ourselves and invite all our friends from our Sunday school class at Park View Mennonite Church, many of them also septuagenarians or soon to be.

Old Massanutten Lodge located east of Keezletown became the perfect setting. The Great Room with massive stone fireplace and stairways leading to a second-story walkway framed by banisters was aglow with seventy votive candles in glass holders when our forty guests arrived.

The dining room table held a bowl of garden roses and three birthday cakes, a favorite for each woman. Ann chose angel food with pineapple icing; Miriam chose German chocolate with coconut pecan frosting; and I chose old-fashioned pound cake with a lemon glaze. A huge cut glass bowl of fresh fruit in an orange glaze, nuts, chips, and beverages completed the display.

We requested that our friends bring no gifts or cards. Instead, we asked them to make a donation to Bridge of Hope, a newly forming ministry for single mothers who were homeless or in danger of becoming homeless. The birthday gift box received nearly eight hundred dollars for this agency.

A choral tribute written by Jay and sung to the tune of "My Country, 'Tis of Thee" began the evening. My verse rang:

> Twins' mom and grandma thrice,
> Cookbooks and quilts suffice
> for leisure roles.
> Work isn't Peggy's fear:
> Sew, plan, or volunteer,
> Help Park View write its mission clear
> and meet its goals.

The program that followed was titled "Songs and Ideas That Speak to Us." Each woman chose a song, selections from her readings, and another woman to offer a prayer or blessing. My song was the American folk melody "How Firm a Foundation" with words of promise "I'll strengthen thee, help thee, and cause thee to stand, upheld by my righteous, omnipotent hand . . ." These are words that had often assured me during times of fear or "fiery trial."

My readings were the poem "Handles" written by Jay about my grandmother's cups and saucers and a selection from the novel, *Hannah Coulter*, written by Wendell Berry (Shoemaker and Hoard, 2004).

Hannah Coulter, also a seventy-year-old woman, reflects on her life:

> And so Nathan required me to think a thought that has stayed with me a long time and has traveled a long way. It passed through everything I know and changed it all. The chance you had is the life you've got. You can make complaints about what people, including you, make of their lives after they have got them and about what people make of other people's lives, even about your children being gone, but you mustn't wish for another life. You mustn't want to be somebody else. What you must do is this: "Rejoice evermore. Pray without ceasing. In everything, give thanks." I am not all the way capable of so much, but those are the right instructions. (p. 113.)

My friend and a former pastor, Shirley Yoder Brubaker, gave me this blessing based on Psalm 92: 12-14:

> May the fruit of your tree be pleasing,
> May your roots grow long and deep,
> May your branches reach toward heaven,
> And your shade cover those in want.
> Amen.

The orange glaze on our bowl of fresh fruit was from my collection. It has been requested numerous times, and I am happy to share it with all. In this way, each user becomes a part of my birthday celebration!

FRESH FRUIT WITH ORANGE GLAZE

1 cup sugar
2 tablespoons plus 1 teaspoon cornstarch
1 cup orange juice
½ cup water
¼ cup lemon juice
½ teaspoon grated orange peel
¼ teaspoon grated lemon peel

Eight cups assorted fresh fruits in season (Peaches, blueberries, pineapple, and bananas are a delicious combination.)

Slices of kiwi or sprigs of fresh peppermint

1. In a small saucepan, combine the sugar and cornstarch. Stir in the orange juice, water, lemon juice, and orange and lemon peels until blended. Bring to a boil; cook and stir for two minutes or until thickened.
2. Cover and refrigerate until chilled.
3. Fold into fresh fruit; garnish and serve. Yield: two cups of glaze; ten servings.

ANTIQUING

The first antiques I ever owned were the blue-and-white cups and saucers without handles that were willed to me by my grandmother Heatwole. These I treasure.

After that, other relatives thought they could make me into a collector of cups and saucers by giving them to me as birthday gifts or on other occasions. Great Aunt Nettie even crocheted me a yellow and green set and starched it stiff to stand on its own. But owning a collection doesn't make one a collector. Love does that. Over time, though, these cup-and-saucer gifts have taken on some significance because of the givers. Some remind me of Granddaddy Suter who gave me several as birthday gifts.

The Valley Pike or Route 11, north and south of Harrisonburg, is host to dozens of small shops and larger antique malls. Jay and I discovered their charm sometime after the girls had established their own homes, and we had time on Sunday afternoons for short getaways. We meandered over the mountain east to Ruckersville, over the mountain west to Franklin, north on Eleven to Strasburg, and south to Lexington with several stops on each trip.

"Look at this," we'd say. "We had one like this when I was a child. Wonder whatever happened to it." Or "Someone gave us a cookie jar like this for a wedding gift, but we sold it later at a yard sale. A shame—look what it's worth now." Or "We have a vase just like this, but we didn't pay nearly this much for it!" Occasionally, we'd say, "Come over here and look." That usually meant that an object of interest had been spotted!

Cobalt blue glassware is not hard to spot. Its deep blue tones are as immediately apparent to the modern collector as they were to the Mycenaeans who produced cobalt blue around 1400 BC. In ancient times, men discovered that a small amount of cobalt, an ore similar in appearance to silver, could be added in the glass-making process to turn the glass into a deep blue.

During the Depression Era, the Hazel Atlas Company produced the most well-known lines of cobalt blue glass. The company began production of its Royal Lace pattern in 1934 and continued until 1941. Its delicate, intricate design made it a popular pattern for collectors, which we became. We now own more than eighty pieces, enough to set a pretty table for our guests. In the end, I have become a collector of certain cups and saucers but only after I fell in love with these blue ones.

I must confess that our cobalt "finds" have not been limited to Royal Lace. Numerous pieces of Mount Pleasant tableware, vases of about every shape and size, children's mugs and toys, oil lamps, peanut jar, covered compote, candy dishes, and more have found their way into our cupboards and onto our shelves.

I further confess that our collection of antiques has not been limited to cobalt blue items. Pieces of furniture and dishes once owned by our grandparents, silver napkin rings, Great Aunt Maude's baby shoes and the peanut lamp we found in her attic, Grandma Landis's market basket, the *Harmonia Sacra* published in 1860, and other treasures reside in our keeping.

There are folks who adopt stray animals and give them a good home. We adopt aging artifacts and try to give them a good home while they are in our care. In many ways, these artifacts do not belong to us. We are simply their stewards as they make their journeys on into the future.

Once in a while, the *Inglenook Cook Book,* first published by the Brethren Publishing House, Elgin, Illinois, in 1911, turns up in an antique shop. Jay found one from the first reprinting in 1970 and gave it to me as a gift. I have selected the recipe for ham potpie to include here. I have never actually used this recipe and probably will not serve it, but it evokes the memory of this salty, old-fashioned dish that my mother used to make with the broth from a leftover ham bone and her homemade noodles.

HAM POTPIE

Take a ham bone after the meat is pretty well used, then boil till tender. Slice two or three good-sized potatoes. Take out the ham bone and put in the potatoes. Let cook while making dumplings. Take about three pints of flour, a pinch of salt, and a rounding tablespoon of shortening, mix together with water. Roll out as thin as pie crust. Cut in any desired shape and drop into the broth with a sprinkle of black pepper.

—Sister M. C. Whitesel, Wayside, Wash. (p. 64, 65)

B

\'bē\ (also b)
n. (pl. bs or b's)
the second letter of the alphabet

BOOKS AND READING

Recipe: Applesauce Cake

Recipe: Raspberry Cream Cheese Cake

BOOKS AND READING

"Tell me a story" was an appeal to Mother that was easily granted, even when she was clipping laundry to the clothesline to dry in the sun or punching down bread dough for its second rising. When my brother and I were very young, she opened her memory book of *Mother Goose Rhymes* and invited us to say them with her. "Jack and Jill went up the hill to fetch a pail of water," we chanted, followed by "Little Bo Peep" who lost her sheep and all the others we could remember. We needed no picture book because we had a cistern on our farm where Jack and Jill could pump their pail of water, and our wooly sheep birthed wobbly lambs every spring. How terrible to lose them!

When we were a little older, the nursery rhymes were replaced by a dozen or so longer story poems that Mother recited from memory. One favorite was "The Green Mountain Justice."

"The snow is deep," the Justice said;
There's mighty mischief overhead . . .
So hand me up the spade, my dear,
I'll mount the barn, the roof to clear."

The wife, afraid her husband would "slip and fall and die," agreed to tie one end of the rope around her waist and the other around his. When the Justice did slip, neither died, but each was left swinging halfway up and halfway down. This one-hundred-line story in rhyming couplets comprised the perfect mix of humor and suspense, and we asked for it so often that eventually I could recite it myself.

The Newberry Medal for distinguished children's books was first given in 1922, and the Caldecott Medal for picture books followed in 1938. Both predate my birth, but I never met the early award winners when I was a child. Our small bookcase held few children's books, but even so, I do not feel impoverished by a lack of stories.

In 1946, I entered the first grade. Those mysterious combinations of my ABCs were unlocked for me by Dick and Jane, their mother and father, and their pets, Spot and Puff, as I was called each day by my teacher to join the circle of low wooden chairs beside her desk. I learned their sounds, and they became words. Words in combination became stories. Stories became information, inspiration, and escape to new worlds of the imagination.

In the second grade, my teacher gave each student one of the books that were being discarded from the all-school library. Mine was a small red-bound volume entitled *Little Black Sambo* that told the enchanting story of a clever little African lad who tricked the jealous tigers into chasing each other around a palm tree until they became butter for his pancakes!

One day during third grade, my teacher needed to leave the room for a short while. (These were the days before tort insurance was necessary, I presume!) She asked me to read stories aloud to my classmates until she returned, so apparently, my reading skills were developing well enough to make that possible.

At home, Mother was reading books aloud to us before bedtime. The *Five Little Peppers* series (copyright, 1918 by Harriet Lothrop) told the story of five children living in dire circumstances following the death of their father. When it was time to celebrate Mamsie's birthday, they worked against the odds to find enough brown flour, cinnamon, and raisins to bake a cake for her, only to have the old oven burn the top of their cake black, a tragedy they remedied with a wreath of flowers.

Christmas 1947, my cousins, Stanley, Shirley, and Janet Suter, gave me a copy of *Heidi* by Johanna Spyri. The two things I remember most vividly from this story are the slice of goat cheese which the grandfather toasted over the fire on the prongs of a long iron fork and the whistling sound of the Alpine winds in the fir trees outside Heidi's hayloft window. Sensory details undoubtedly made these settings come alive to me.

Laura Ingalls Wilder (1867-1957) wrote the series of eight *Little House* books, describing the difficult life of her family as they homesteaded on the plains. Not only a transport for the pioneer spirit in me and my brother and every child, these stories also provided invaluable character-building lessons. How can I forget the endurance and perseverance of Father as he stretched a clothesline from the house to the barn to feel his way through the blinding blizzard to feed his animals?

Daddy owned several of the popular adventure novels of Zane Grey (1872-1939) that presented an idealized image of the Old West. Western fiction such as *Riders of the Purple Sage* and *The Thundering Herd* were certainly not written for little girls, but I read them anyway, totally immersed in the struggle between valiant men and villains, their horses, and the brave Navajo warriors that often rode in just in time to aid in the rescue. The language in these novels reflected the rugged life of the characters, and once when I was called from my reading to hoe thistles in the afternoon sun, the swear words buzzed through my head like bees!

In time, I moved into the dreamy land of the romance novel and borrowed numerous versions of essentially the same story by Grace Livingston Hill from our small church library. Zane Grey and Grace Livingston Hill represented a pendulum swing (too rough and too smooth), but a better reading balance was finally achieved when I discovered books such as *Gone with the Wind* by Margaret Mitchell and *Jane Eyre* by Charlotte Bronte.

This recipe for applesauce cake is adapted from my mother's file. It has the potential to be more flavorful than the simple cake baked by the Five Little Peppers, but it is of the same nutritious vintage and can be baked with just as much love!

APPLESAUCE CAKE

½ cup butter
1 cup light brown sugar
2 eggs, well beaten
1 and ½ cups applesauce
2 cups unbleached, all-purpose flour
1 teaspoon soda (dissolved in the applesauce)
1 teaspoon baking powder
½ teaspoon cinnamon
½ teaspoon nutmeg
⅛ teaspoon cloves
1 teaspoon vanilla
I cup raisins
½ cup chopped walnuts (optional)

1. Cream shortening and sugar and beat until fluffy.
2. Add eggs and combine thoroughly.
3. Add half of the applesauce and soda mixture and blend. Sift dry ingredients and add alternately with remaining applesauce. Add vanilla.
4. Fold raisins and nuts into the batter.
5. Pour into a greased and lightly floured loaf pan, five by nine by four inches.
6. Bake at 350 degrees for fifty minutes until toothpick comes out clean.
7. Cool for ten minutes in pan before turning onto wire rack.

During the college and career years, my reading ran along practical lines. I read constantly, but most was in order to complete class assignments, keep up with educational trends, renew my teacher's certificate, and find solutions to work problems I encountered. Some of this reading was also delightful, especially my reading for classes in children's literature and adolescent fiction.

At times, I was able to blend work and pleasure. My eighth grade English classes studied *Shane* by Jack Schaefer (1949), one of the most popular westerns of all time. The mysterious Shane rode to the rescue of Wyoming homesteaders, a nobleman on horseback. Here was a cleaned-up version of my earlier Zane Grey novels, enjoyed as much by teacher as students.

The two best travel guides I ever read were *The Source* by James Michener (1965), and *Trinity* by Leon Uris (1976). *The Source* covers the scope of Israeli history as each new archaeological level of a tel is excavated, while *Trinity* chronicles Northern Irish families from 1840 to 1916. Visits to each of these countries, soon after reading the book, made what I was seeing even more meaningful.

In 1992, in a London bookstore, I picked up a copy of Jane Smiley's recent winner of the Pulitzer Prize for Fiction, *A Thousand Acres,* in which she transposes the tragedy of King Lear to a modern-day setting in Iowa. This influenced my goal for the six-month hiatus I was to have between two careers—to read all the Pulitzer winners of the last ten years. These included *Lonesome Dove* (1986) by Larry McMurtry (more Zane Grey!), two "Rabbit" winners by John Updike (1982 and 1991), and *Breathing Lessons* (1989) by Anne Tyler whose colorful character portrayals I have loved in many of her novels since.

Reading has often enhanced and guided my meditation. The stand alone in this category will always be *The Psalms* of the Old Testament. How many times has God reminded me that "his love endures forever" (Psalm 107:1) or that I may "cast my cares on the Lord, and he will sustain me (Psalm 55:22)? These and other poetic promises have nurtured me in every difficult experience of my life.

Frequently, one sees a top ten list of best sellers. Here are my "Top Ten Best Devotional Books," alphabetically by author:

Buechner, Frederick, *Listening to Your Life,* Harper Collins, 1992.

Buechner, Frederick, *The Sacred Journey,* Harper & Row, 1982.

Daily Light on the Daily Path, Harper and Row, 1950.

(This book was given to me in 1963 by Arlene Bumbaugh, a very special teacher, neighbor, and friend with the inscription, "To Peggy, with love, when Ann and Jill came to live with the Landises.")

Foster, Richard J., *Celebration of Discipline,* Harper & Row, 1978.

Julian of Norwich Showings, Paulist Press, 1978.

Kropf, Marlene, and Eddy Hall, *Praying with the Anabaptists,* Faith and Life Press, 1994.

L'Engle, Madeleine, *A Circle of Quiet,* The Seabury Press, 1972.

Merton, Thomas, *The Seven Storey Mountain,* Harcourt Brace, 1948.

Norris, Kathleen, *Amazing Grace: A Vocabulary of Faith,* Riverhead Books, 1998.

Palmer, Parker, *The Active Life: A Spirituality of Work, Creativity, and Caring,* Harper & Row, 1990.

The Eastern Mennonite College Faculty Ladies Book Club began sometime in the early 1960s as one of several social groups available to female employees and female spouses of employees. I was a member in those early days but became too busy with my young family and career to keep up with meetings.

Much has changed since that time. The Book Club, as it is now known, is no longer an extension of the university, and members do not refer to themselves as "ladies," rather as "women." Ruth Lehman was one of the charter members and for many years was the "bookkeeper" of the group. She faithfully kept record of all the books and authors the club read.

At Ruth's invitation, I rejoined the club in the early 1990s after I resigned from my last full-time job. Although the name had changed, I was happy to find that many things remained the same. The group is comprised of women who meet on the first Monday night of each month in a member's home. We sit in a circle. We select upcoming books from recommendations of group members. We wait until "the price comes down" even when that prevents us from reading a new book for a little longer. We select a discussion leader, usually from the group, but everyone pitches in as soon as the invitation is extended. Finally, we end the evening with a delicious dessert and beverage and informal visiting.

I appreciate my association with this group of approximately twenty-five women, mostly in retirement. Their keen minds and wide-ranging experiences spark many stimulating discussions. I have read books I would not have selected myself, only to discover another culture or current topic of great interest.

A whole cookbook of decadent desserts could be compiled by the members of the Book Club. Of those recipes, none would top Ruby Lehman's signature peach pie! I once served raspberry cheese cake which met the group's approval. It is delicious!

RASPBERRY CREAM CHEESE CAKE

CAKE:
2 and ¼ cups all-purpose flour
¾ cup sugar
¾ cup cold butter
½ teaspoon baking powder
½ teaspoon baking soda
¾ cup sour cream
1 egg, beaten
1 and ½ teaspoons almond extract

FILLING:
1 package (8 ounces) cream cheese, softened
½ cup sugar

1 egg
½ cup raspberry jam
½ cup slivered almonds

1. Combine flour and sugar; cut in butter until mixture is crumbly. Set aside one cup. Add baking powder, soda, salt, sour cream, egg, and almond extract to the remaining mixture and mix well. Spread into the bottom and two inches up the side of a greased nine-inch springform pan.
2. Combine cream cheese, sugar, and egg; beat well. Spoon over batter. Top with raspberry jam, reserved crumb mixture, and slivered almonds. Bake at 350 degrees for fifty-five to sixty minutes. Cool on wire rack for fifteen minutes before removing sides of pan. Cool completely and store in refrigerator.

> (Adapted from *Taste of Home's Complete Guide to Baking*,
> Taste of Home Books, 2004.)

In conclusion to this chapter about books and reading, I must add that I love to read cookbooks! I can always enjoy an hour with *Complete Guide to Baking* which was a gift from my dear friend, Irene Mullenex.

C \'sē\ (also c)
n. (pl. cs or c's)
the third letter of the alphabet

CHICAGO AVENUE

Recipe: Arlene's Potato Soup

CHRISTMAS

Recipe: Medium Dark Fruitcake

Recipe: Oyster Dressing

COVENTRY CATHEDRAL

Recipe: Split Pea Soup with Barley

CHICAGO AVENUE

The Chicago Avenue Mennonite Church of the early 1940s and the Coventry Cathedral of another entry were vastly dissimilar. To suggest a comparison between a world renowned cathedral and a tiny church plant may be ludicrous. However, both were houses of Christian worship, both were impacted to greater or lesser degrees by war, and both taught a doctrine of reconciliation and peacemaking. Both are part of my religious experience.

Chicago Avenue began in 1936 when students from the YPCA (Young People's Christian Association) of Eastern Mennonite College began a Sunday school in an unused restaurant in Harrisonburg. A year later, they rented a small white church building on the corner of Chicago Avenue and Green Streets for fifteen dollars a month. Within three years, the property was purchased for three thousand dollars; and in 1946, it was officially recognized as a congregation by Virginia Mennonite Conference.

Our family and others began to attend Chicago Avenue during the war when gas rationing kept us from driving a greater distance. My parents liked the small intimate circle of friends they made there, the inclusive atmosphere, and the more progressive direction the congregation was taking.

The church building at that time was very small, with an assembly area seating less than one hundred people. Steps led to a basement where a few children's classrooms were located. I remember being dismissed after the opening songs of the Sunday evening service to go to the basement for Bible quizzes, spelldowns of memory verses, and rousing songs with motions ("This little light of mine, I'm going to let it shine—all over Harrisonburg!"). Sometimes a returned missionary would talk to us about people on a faraway continent. Other times, we were entertained with flannel board stories.

The church was the primary locus of our family's social life. We attended at least three times a week—Sunday morning preaching and Sunday school, Sunday evening young people's meeting, and Wednesday evening prayer meeting. Each summer, there was a two-week Vacation Bible School, which was no vacation for my mother who always taught a class and managed to keep up with our garden as well. Folks invited other families home for fried chicken dinners after church. There were potlucks and picnics, mission projects, boys and girls clubs, youth group meetings, sewing circles, and song services.

I was baptized at Chicago Avenue when I was twelve years old following a response I had made during summertime tent revival meetings held by Brother Kenneth Good. The bishop of our district, Daniel W. Lehman, conducted instruction classes for several months for me and others who wished to become members of the church. He even made one home visit to each person where he tested our Bible knowledge and our understanding of the important step we were taking. He told my mother that he was more than satisfied with my answers.

On the Sunday morning of my baptism, I was nervous and self-conscious. I was wearing the white net prayer covering for the first time. When Brother Daniel uncupped his hands, the water ran down my face as I kneeled forward with head bowed for my baptism. I was then extended "the right hand of fellowship" and challenged to "walk in newness of life." Sisters of the church (ministers' and deacons' wives) came forward to greet me with "the holy kiss." With this solemn ritual, I became a lifelong member of the Mennonite church.

Chicago Avenue gave me my earliest experiences in leadership when I became president of the MYF (Mennonite Youth Fellowship). I remember writing agendas for our cabinet meetings that I conducted at the dining room table of my home. I learned the importance of working with others to implement plans. Youth sponsors such as Ken and June Marie Weaver and Evelyn and Shelly Wenger became my mentors.

The guiding light for these formative years was our pastor, Brother Harold G. Eshleman. He was a strong leader, demanding and deserving the respect of Chicago Avenue's members. Weekdays, he was an elementary teacher and principal in Rockingham County Public Schools; evenings and weekends, he nurtured his congregation, and if any time remained, he ministered to the needs of immigrants and the neglected in the community. His wife, Arlene, a trained secretary and a fantastic cook, kept her husband organized and maintained a sense of humor about the "Billy Wrights" who frequently showed up for supper. I know this because I too frequently showed up for a meal—as the guest of their daughter, Ruth, who was one of my best friends.

Here is Arlene Eshleman's recipe for potato soup. She may have served this with a golden round of Colby cheese and crackers or a sandwich spread made from Lebanon bologna. Pie would have been a likely dessert. When I make this soup, I sometimes add tiny florets of broccoli that I microwave for one minute and put into the soup just before serving. It adds a bit of color and maybe a few extra vitamins.

ARLENE'S POTATO SOUP

1/3 cup chopped celery
⅓ cup chopped onion
2 tablespoons butter
4 cups peeled, diced potatoes
3 cups chicken broth
2 cups milk
1 teaspoon salt
¼ teaspoon pepper
Dash of paprika
2 cups shredded cheddar cheese

1. In a saucepan, sauté celery and onion in margarine until tender.
2. Add potatoes and broth. Cover and simmer until potatoes are tender, about twelve minutes. Puree in blender or mash with potato masher (allow a few chunks to remain).
3. Stir in milk, salt, pepper, and paprika.
4. When very hot, add cheese and heat until melted. Makes about eight servings.

CHRISTMAS

The approaching Christmas season was her *raison d'etre* for stopping at Woolworth's candy counter each time she went shopping after Thanksgiving. The glass cases displayed all the sweet treats inside—orange slices, nonpareils, Mary Janes, little white and pink coconut squares, Jordan almonds, peanut clusters, chocolate-covered raisins, and hard candy to hold in your cheek for a long time. Each time she stopped, she bought a pound or half a pound of this one and that one. The clerk scooped out the chosen candies and poured them onto the scale, all the time watching the red needle and deciding whether to drop yet one more or perhaps remove a piece. When Mother got home, she hid the little brown bags in the wooden chest in her bedroom. Later, she used her stash to make candy dishes displaying the tantalizing variety.

In the weeks before Christmas, other preparations were also under way. At school, I learned to sing:
"Up on the housetop—click, click, click,
Down through the chimney with good Saint Nick."
We made Santas with red construction paper suits and cotton ball beards. Children gave each other small presents—little cobalt bottles of Evening in Paris eau de cologne, embroidered handkerchiefs, paper dolls, or ceramic animals. My first grade boyfriend, Norman, gave me a tiny tea set made of white porcelain. I played with it for many years and still have one small cup and saucer.

I willingly gave my imagination to Santa Claus but my heart to the Baby Jesus, whose birthday I knew we *really* were celebrating. At church, we sang "Away in a Manger" and had a Sunday evening program where every child had a "part." Sometimes I spoke the "welcome recitation" or read the narration for the reenactment of the Nativity. Each time, Mother coached me to say it "with expression." Every year, we children waited eagerly for the conclusion of the program when all would receive a gift. We knew exactly what it would be and would have been sorely disappointed if it had been anything different. Those orange mesh stockings filled with nuts and candy, peppermint cane, and tangerine were all any Sunday school child could hope for at Christmastime!

All Daddy's siblings, their spouses, and their children gathered around Grandma Heatwole's table in the years before her death. The jovial, noisy crowd feasted on the best foods of their tradition and ended the evening with a giant gift exchange where every family gave a gift to every child in all the other families. As the evening wore on, I became tired and grouchy. When I received a set of toy cooking implements identical to a set I had opened some minutes before, I forgot my manners completely and said petulantly,

"I'm didn't want two dippers." (How many times did Mother remind me of her embarrassment?)

The Suter family couldn't gather under one roof because Aunt Helen and her family lived in Maryland, and a wintertime trip just wasn't feasible. Each year, Aunt Helen sent her Christmas box by Parcel Post. For days, we eagerly waited for the mail carrier to deliver this mysteriously wonderful package which contained a gift for each and a generous sample of Aunt Helen's homemade fudge!

Granddaddy Suter delighted each of his eleven grandchildren with the extravagantly generous gift of five dollars every year! We expected it, looked forward to it, and began planning how we would spend it long before December arrived. It was thrilling to be so wealthy once each year, especially during those post-World War II years.

The week before Christmas, our family put on boots and tramped all over the hill behind the barn where cedar and juniper trees grew wild. "Not that one. It's too tall," Daddy would say. "This one is crooked." "The cows have rubbed against this one, and one side is bare." Then finally, "Here's a good one! See how green it is, how straight and bushy!" Then he chopped it down, and we dragged it home to be erected in a bucket of stones in the living room. We decorated it simply with a string of lights, some shiny balls and the tinsel we saved from year to year. Always the aromatic fragrance of the cedar far outdid the tree's visual grandeur.

Presents didn't arrive under the tree until Jimmy and I had gone to bed on Christmas Eve. With wakeful anticipation, we heard the rustlings in our parents' bedroom closet and the screen door bump as Daddy brought in something from the outside.

One year, I was doing a little snooping but hadn't found much when Mother caught me looking into her bedroom closet. "That box is mine," she told me firmly as she ushered me out of the room.

On Christmas morning, Jimmy and I got up very early and went to the tree to discover our presents. That box was there, but I didn't open it; it was Mother's present, I remembered. A little later, we climbed onto our parents' bed to talk about our presents. "Did you like your doll?" Mother asked. With unveiled disappointment, I said that I did not get a doll. "Go back and look in that box," Mother said. "But it's yours," I reminded her. "It *was* mine until I gave it to you," she told me.

I lifted the lid, and there was my pretty doll with eyes that opened and closed.

I have in my possession page 28 from the December 1954 issue of *The Southern Planter*, one of the few magazines that came regularly to our rural mailbox. The page is yellowed and broken along the crease lines from years of use. There are several brown splotches on one side.

Peggy H. Landis

The page tells the story of how Mrs. Hall's home economics classes in Henrico County, Virginia, baked fruitcakes each year and sold them to benefit the FHA (Future Homemakers of America) of Varina High School. Herein lies the special recipe Mother used every November to bake the fruitiest, most moist and spicy cakes ever pulled from an oven.

Mother usually doubled the recipe in order to bake gifts for neighbors and friends. She always saved some of the almond slivers and candied cherries to decorate the top of each cake. After the cakes were baked and cooled, she wrapped them loosely in old linen tea towels and sealed them along with apples halves in lard cans to "age."

Do not dare to joke about fruitcakes until you have had a slice of this with your cup of tea!

MEDIUM DARK FRUITCAKE

12 eggs, separated
1 pound sugar
1 pound seedless raisins
1 pound butter
½ pound citron, diced
½ pound almonds, blanched and cut fine
1 pound currants, washed and fried
½ pound black walnuts, chopped
½ pound candied cherries, cut in half
¼ pound lemon peel, cut fine
¼ pound orange peel, cut fine
1 four-ounce package figs, cut fine
1 package dates, cut fine
1 teaspoon each cinnamon, cloves, and nutmeg
½ teaspoon allspice
2 pounds flour
1 cup light molasses or syrup
½ teaspoon soda, mix in syrup
1 cup orange juice
2 cups diced candied pineapple

Cream butter, add sugar, and beat until light and fluffy. Add egg yolks and beat well. Combine fruits and nuts. Sift over flour which has been sifted with dry ingredients. Mix well. Add floured fruits to first mixture alternately with molasses (to which soda has been added) and orange juice. Mix well and fold in stiffly beaten egg whites. Pour in two large tube cake pans which have been greased and lined with waxed paper or five small loaf pans. Bake large cakes at 275 degrees for three to four hours. Smaller cakes take one and a half to two hours. This recipe makes ten pounds of fruitcake.

Counting our courtship years, Jay and I have spent well over fifty happy Christmases together. We had dated only a few months before Christmas 1957 when I was eighteen, and he was seven years my senior. Would he give me a gift, I wondered. What should I give him in return?

He gave me a little poetry book by Alfred Noyes, *Daddy Fell into the Pond* (Sheed and Ward, 1952). During the holidays, Aunt Alice asked whether my boyfriend had given me a gift. "Yes," I answered, "a book of poetry." "What is the title?" she queried. With a little hesitation, I replied, *"Daddy Fell into the Pond."* Her eyes suggested what my heart feared, that he thought of me as a child or at best a young student.

In the next years, he completely redeemed himself (or I grew up) with gifts the likes of a trip to New York City and a piano—more than enough to meet Aunt Alice's approval!

Over time, the gifts of poetry were bumped up quite a few notches as well. Christmas 1977, he wrote this sonnet for me:

Peggy's Canticle

I offer you my own magnificat—
You too are highly favored, and the Lord
Is with you. Countless gabriel-sendings dot
Your nazareth landscapes, hailings richly stored
To ponder quietly. For abraham
And latent generations mercy flows—
A trusted root twice sprung at bethlehem.
I praise, your children bless, the virtuous rose,
Our mary-one, whose ministry expands
In understandings, knowings, listenings (hearts
Made light), and writings, sewings, cookings (hands
Made glad). Such endless newnesses impart
Yourself, I would like chosen joseph glow,
Honored—because of you—magnifico.

When Ann and Jill were very little and messily eating Gerber's baby food by the carton, Jay and I had dozens of the little glass jars at our disposal. Borrowing an idea from some publication, we created a glass Christmas tree by filling the jars with water of several colors and stacking them in a tall tier. A string of lights wrapped around a dowel stick in the center sparkled through the water for a dazzling effect.

One year, I used a McCalls pattern and fabric scraps from my stash to create a menagerie of Winnie the Pooh animals for our little preschool girls. Playful Tigger was fashioned from orange fabric marked with felt-tip stripes. Navy blue Eeyore had long floppy ears and a very dour expression. Piglet, the baby pig, wore a little blue shirt over his pale pink body while brown mother Kanga carried Baby Roo proudly in her pocket. Most loveable of all was Pooh himself, a yellow bear in a charming red shirt.

Jill and Ann made Christmas tree ornaments in elementary school that become greater treasures as they become ever shabbier with time. Jill crafted a gold-felt stocking that she stuffed with cotton before stitching the edges in green. Her initials "J. L." are embroidered boldly in the center. Ann's ornament is a small Nativity scene. Inside the brown construction paper is a paper Mary and Joseph stand behind the manger with tiny blades of yellow straw glued painstakingly in place.

Several Christmases were spent in Idaho away from family and close friends. Handmade Christmas cards became our means of connection. One year, I carved four "head shapes," representing each of us, from potatoes, and we sat around our small kitchen table all afternoon stamping our images onto our greetings. On the bottom back, we labeled each card "A Genuine Idaho Potato Print!"

For many years, we gathered at Mother's house on Christmas Day along with Uncle Jim and Aunt Ruby, Keith, and Kim. Everyone brought gifts for Grandma, and she gave us hers, often handcrafted, such as the gigantic fleece pillows she made to watch television while lying on the floor. The highlight of the day was always her dinner, beautifully served on a lace cloth over green. The food was sumptuous—country ham, fried oysters or oyster dressing, many vegetables and side dishes, and finally fresh coconut cake, fruit salad, and a tray of homemade candies and fruitcake.

Then the scenery shifted, and Grandma brought her dish of oyster dressing and sat at our table with our children and grandchildren. New traditions developed.

One favorite tradition has been Christmas crackers, an idea we brought back from our semesters in England. "Crackers" or "poppers," as three-year-old Becky chose to call them, are made by wrapping small gifts inside a two-by-four-inch cylinder covered with wrapping paper and tied at the ends with ribbon. We customize our crackers by attaching a personal rhyme or riddle with a hint of the contents inside. The crackers are placed on the table with the dessert, and in turn, each person tries to guess what is inside before pulling the ends to crack it open.

One year, the Sniders purchased gifts for everyone from the Broadway Ben Franklin store. My cracker contained a two-and-a-half-inch measuring square for my quilting projects. Their clever rhyme read:

Some would quibble at being called square,
But it's needed when piecing a quilt.
Mom can quonnect the quorners just right;
She qualified, quareful, and skill't.

My journal entry on Christmas Eve 2008 reveals other traditions and delights of the season. "Jay brought in greens for me to use in decorating the house . . . One of the lovely surprises of the day was a gift he asked me to open early—a Nativity dome under which a burning votive candle creates stars. I had admired it in a store earlier and had no idea he had bought it . . . Rachael, who lives in our apartment, brought us a loaf of her yeasty multigrain bread and a container of honey cinnamon butter . . . About 3:30 p.m., Ann and Sue arrived from Tallahassee—and Bunchie and Casey—so we sat down and had a cup of coffee and the biscotti that Kate, our neighbor across the street, had brought. As usual the candlelight Christmas Eve service at church was crowded, and people were saving seats for family. The Sniders joined the rest of us on the bench. Jay sang in the choir, and the congregation sang a lot of carols, including the beautiful "Star of Bethlehem."

OYSTER DRESSING

6 to 8 cups dried bread, cut into one-inch cubes
¼ cup finely chopped celery
2 tablespoons finely chopped onion
1 pint standard size oysters, liquor reserved
salt and pepper to taste
5 eggs, beaten
3 and ½ cups milk
3 tablespoons melted butter
2 tablespoons fresh parsley, chopped

Spread half the bread cubes in a greased 9x12 baking dish. Add the celery and onion. Distribute the oysters evenly over the dish and sprinkle with salt and pepper. Top with remaining bread crumbs. Mix beaten eggs, milk, and reserved oyster liquor and pour evenly over the crumbs. Drizzle melted butter over the top.

Bake at 350 degrees for approximately fifty minutes or until golden on top and not "juicy" in the middle. Sprinkle with chopped parsley and serve immediately.

COVENTRY CATHEDRAL

One Sunday morning in 1997, we and our group of students left Stratford, England, in our coach and motored to the city of Coventry in the West Midlands. *En route,* our tour guide, Robert Stanyon, told us how World War II had affected the lives of the British people. He was a young child at the time, and he recalled his own experience of being sent by train from his home in London. Robert and many other children, wearing wooden tags with their names and destination, were sent to Cambridge to wait until the war ended. Robert's mother was a pharmacist, considered essential personnel, and not allowed to accompany him.

How little I know about war! I was a small child during World War II, and my father had a military deferment. I have a very shadowy memory of a nighttime siren when we turned off all our lights and another dim memory of the ration books with stamps for sugar and gasoline. The subsequent wars with Korea, Vietnam, Afghanistan, and Iraq were fought on foreign soils, and although modern media have brought pictures of their horrors to our house, I have not suffered physically. I did not choose the era of my existence or my location on the planet; I can only wonder at my privilege.

On November 14, 1940, when I was only three months old, the industrial city of Coventry in central England was reduced to rubble by the German Luftwaffe. Saint Michael's Cathedral, begun in the thirteenth century and one of the largest parish churches in England, burned with the city. Only the tower, outer walls, spire, and crypt survived. On the following morning, the decision to rebuild was announced, not as an act of defiance, but as a sign of faith and hope for the future.

Sir Basil Spence was chosen in 1950 as the architect for the new Coventry Cathedral. He insisted that instead of rebuilding the old cathedral, it would be kept in ruins as a garden of remembrance and that a new cathedral should be built beside it, forming one church. The new cathedral was consecrated in May 1962.

With an hour before the beginning of the 10:30 a.m. service, I walked up the steps of the majestic porch, pausing to observe *Saint Michael's Victory over the Devil,* a sculpture by Sir Jacob Epstein, on the outer wall of the new cathedral. Inside the plaza, I took the steps to the left and entered the shell of the once beautiful Gothic cathedral. Almost immediately, my attention turned to the east end where a simple cross of charred timbers stood, a replica of the two wooden beams the cathedral stonemason found lying in the shape of a cross after the firestorm.

Later, young German volunteers worked alongside their English counterparts to clear the rubble. Together, they decided to inscribe some words on the stone wall behind the charred cross. First, they planned to inscribe "Father, forgive them for they know not what they do," but that was too long for the space. Then they agreed to write only, "Father, forgive them." Before the work was done, however, one of the English workers asked that it be shortened even further, so that blame would not fall on any single group involved in the war. They decided to inscribe only two words: "Father, forgive."

Someone has said, "To walk from the ruins to the new cathedral is to walk from Good Friday to Easter, from the ravages of human nature to the glorious hope of resurrection." (Coventry Cathedral website)

Height, light, and color greeted me as they do to every visitor to the new modernist style cathedral. Height is achieved by the soaring nave pillars. Light enters the huge west window known as the *Screen of Saints and Angels*, a gigantic engraving on glass in expressionist style by John Hutton. Color is displayed in the beautiful abstract design of the stained glass Baptistery window by John Piper, a symbol of the light of truth breaking through the conflicts of our world. Every area of the cathedral is replete with the work of artists.

The mission of Coventry Cathedral is straightforward and simple—the ministry of reconciliation. On the altar, a large gilded cross contains the original Cross of Nails. The Cross of Nails was made from three medieval nails collected from the ruins of the old cathedral. Three nails from the ruins have now become the symbol of reconciliation in Centers worldwide in sixty different countries.

The stone structures of the old and new Coventry Cathedral reminded me of Jesus's words to the Pharisees when they told him to hush the praises of the crowd on Palm Sunday. "I tell you," he replied, "if they keep quiet, the stones will cry out." (Luke 19: 40 NIV) The stones of Coventry clearly cry out the message of reconciliation to a world of war. The architecture of this place spoke forcefully to my spirit, a strong sermon without words.

A refectory, I have learned, is a dining hall in a monastery or college. The word is from the Latin, *refectio*, meaning a place of refreshment or nourishment. Most cathedrals have a refectory, and we learned to enjoy the inexpensive but delicious soup and crusty bread they serve. This recipe is reminiscent of those hearty lunchtime bowls.

SPLIT PEA SOUP WITH BARLEY

10 cups of water
1 pound dry yellow or green split peas, rinsed and drained, about 2 cups
½ cup regular barley
2 tablespoons instant chicken bouillon granules
1 bay leaf

2 stalks celery, finely chopped
2 medium carrots, finely chopped (1 cup)
1 medium onion, finely chopped (½ cup)
5 ounces cooked ham, chopped (1 cup)
½ teaspoon ground black pepper
Salt to taste

Bring water, split peas, barley, bouillon granules, and bay leaf to boiling. Reduce heat. Simmer, covered for thirty minutes. Stir in celery, carrots, and onion. Return to boiling. Reduce heat. Simmer, covered for thirty additional minutes or until vegetables are tender.

Stir in ham and ½ teaspoon pepper. Cook until ham is heated through. Remove bay leaf. Season to taste. Makes eight (1 and ½ cups) servings.

D

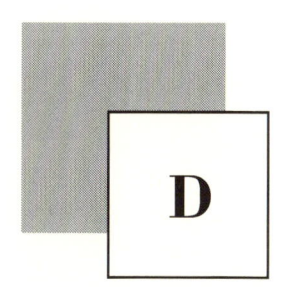

\'dē\ (also d)
n. (pl. ds or d's)
the fourth letter of the alphabet

DADDY

Recipe: Soft Egg Custard

DECLENSIONS AND CONJUGATIONS

Recipe: Chicken and Asparagus Frittata

Recipe: Fried Apples

DADDY

Every life must have its portion of pain. The portion of Daddy's psychiatric pain was so large that it spilled over and brought pain to his wife and children and frequently threatened our home life.

My father, Roy Abram Heatwole (1915-1995), was first hospitalized for treatment at the University of Virginia Medical Center when I was a preschool child. Mother said he was sick and not able to feed the cows. Was he clinically depressed? Was it some psychotic twist? I have never known the diagnosis, and I don't believe Mother could have named it.

The event I remember most from that hospitalization was a trip over the Blue Ridge Mountains with Uncle Frank Swope. He stopped the car at a roadside craft shop where I fell in love with a little black rocking chair for my doll. Uncle Frank said he would buy it for me if I promised to keep it "until I was an old lady." I have kept my promise! When Daddy was released from the hospital, he brought home a little bed he had made for my doll in the woodworking shop.

I was in the fifth grade when I became aware that Daddy was sick again. This episode followed a conflict among his siblings after Grandma Heatwole's death and his disappointment when the homestead was sold outside of the family. Mother called it a "nervous breakdown," and he was hospitalized at DeJarnettes, a stately looking private mental hospital outside of Staunton, Virginia. We went to see him there in a room reserved for visitors, and I remember feeling timid and uncomfortable with him in that unfamiliar place.

Medications and therapy for mentally ill persons were nonexistent or very primitive in the mid-1940s. Daddy received electric shock treatments, a horrible experience he was never willing to talk about, and he vowed he would never again submit to hospital admission. On the day he came home, our family took a walk together over the fields above our barn, but happiness had not returned with him.

In the years that followed, he functioned rather well much of the time and was a successful farmer. In 1951, he bought an eighty-acre farm north of Mount Clinton, Virginia, where he crop farmed, sold A-grade milk, and raised commercial laying hens, stock ewes, lambs, and beef cattle. He loved his animals and took very good care of them.

He believed that he took care of his family too. He was a "good provider," and he never physically abused or hurt any of us. As a teenager, I never asked for money but that he gave it freely, usually accompanied with an injunction to be careful how I spent it or a reminder of how beholden I was to him.

He was always right about everything—even when he was wrong—and he never conceded a point. He was the "head of the household" because the

Bible said so. In fact, he used the Bible as his self-medication, a more positive drug than alcohol, but he distorted its message and used it in judgment on us, the neighbors, the milk company, and the bank if his statement didn't appear to be correct.

Over the years, all the arguments, accusations, and preachments grew to become a raging bonfire and threatened to consume me. When I realized as an adult what my resentment was doing to my spirit, I searched for a way to resolve the inner conflict. To change him was impossible. To find the cause of his behavior was beyond my resources. God didn't answer my prayers.

At last, the simple but difficult answer was given to me—I must forgive him. With a certain amount of peace about this solution, I set out to drop all the suits I had against him and offer him a measure of kindness. There was no magic in this decision, and I learned time after time that forgiveness is not a one-time, easy act but a willingness to try again and again. Although our relationship never became loving, I tried to treat him with respect, realizing that on our best days, neither of us would have chosen the impasse that had developed over the years. I confess too that my own obstinacy and intolerance did nothing to improve the situation.

After he and Mother separated in 1963 and later when he sold the farm and moved to a small house in south Park View, I felt torn on Christmas Day and on other special occasions when the rest of the family gathered without him. I frequently invited him to dinner at my house on Christmas Eve or some alternate time. On these occasions, our daughters enjoyed hearing him talk about his memories of life when he was a boy. Jay became quite adept at steering conversations away from "religion and politics" and other booby traps.

On February 18, 1995, Daddy celebrated his eightieth birthday. A week or so before, I sent postcards to his nieces and nephews and a few neighbors and friends asking them to remember him with a card, if they wished. When he came to our house for dinner on his birthday, he brought the bundle of cards he had received, and his appreciation was clearly evident. My menu attempted to include some of his favorite foods: roast beef, baked corn, and spice cake. He complimented me on my cooking.

In October of the same year, his newspaper carrier told me that he had failed to pick up his paper the previous day. His death was described as a heart attack.

Because of his respect for Bishop Glendon Blosser, we asked him to speak at the memorial service held at Weavers Mennonite Church. He used the Psalms to focus on nature, the earth, and the soil since Daddy had been a farmer and had loved his land, his horses, and his cows; and even in his retirement, he had continued to put out a big garden and tend his marigold beds. The lawn mower was found midrow on the day following his death.

God, in his mercy, took Daddy very suddenly; and in doing so, he spared him and all of us responsible for caring for him in his declining years from further pain and stress.

I look at a picture of Daddy, Mother, and me when I was about three years old. How handsome and tall he stands with thick dark hair, a necktie, and three-pieced suit. His grey eyes are shaded by his prominent brow, but his expression is easy and pleasant. I wonder what tiny aberration—chemical, genetic, or environmental—could have exacted so much struggle from a man who appears so strong.

Among Daddy's papers, I found a handwritten recipe for soft custard which he had requested from his sister, my Aunt Alice, after he lived alone. It appears that she told him how to make it by telephone.

Our farm produced all the milk and eggs we wished to use, and sometimes Mother made this hot eggnog on a cold winter evening after Daddy and Jim came in from the barn. We drank it from mugs while it was still hot—delicious! Add a shake of nutmeg for a spicy flavor enhancement.

SOFT EGG CUSTARD

4 eggs
4 tablespoons sugar
4 cups milk
½ teaspoon vanilla
Nutmeg (optional)

Beat eggs well and mix in sugar. Set aside.

Scald milk in top of a double boiler.

Pour milk slowly into beaten eggs, stirring as you pour.

Transfer milk and eggs back to top of double boiler.

Heat, stirring constantly, until mixture coats a spoon or sounds "soft" when poured from the spoon. Never let the mixture boil!

When mixture begins to thicken, pour immediately through a sieve (to remove any egg "curdles") into a bowl.

Add vanilla.

Sprinkle with nutmeg, if desired.

Custard may be served hot or cold. It is a delicious sauce over apple pie or can be combined with other ingredients in desserts such as graham cracker pudding.

DECLENSIONS AND CONJUGATIONS

As a young lad, Sir Winston Churchill was sent to Harrow, a boarding school for boys located in northwest London. There he met the First Declension of the Latin language.

Nominative	*mensa*	a table
Genitive	*mensae*	of a table
Dative	*mensae*	to or for a table
Accusative	*mensam*	a table (object)
Ablative	*mensa*	by or with a table
Vocative	*mensa*	O Table

When he inquired about the use of the vocative, *mensa,* the don responded that it would be used in addressing a table, as in speaking directly to a table. "But I never do!" was young Winston's impertinent reply.

Because of his unwillingness to learn Latin, he was thought dull and compelled to study only English. In his autobiography, *My Early Life* (Scribner's, 1930), Churchill says that being so long in the lowest form actually gave him an advantage over the clever boys who went on to study Latin and Greek. He learned his English thoroughly. "Naturally, I am biased in favor of boys learning English," he wrote. "I would make them all learn English, and then I would let the clever ones learn Latin as an honor and Greek as a treat. But the only thing I would whip them for is not knowing English; I would whip them hard for that."

I met my first noun of the First Declension, *femina* (woman), and my first verb of the First Conjugation, *porto* (I carry), in the fall of 1956. "Porto, portas, portat, portamus, portatis, portant," I chanted with my classmates until the words sang in our heads for ready reference. During the course of the next four years, I went on to learn the harder things—gerunds and the subjunctive—and to translate bits of Roman literature.

My professor was Dorothy C. Kemrer, a nunlike lady who lived in her cloistered apartment in the southeast corner of the women's dormitory. She was in every way as precise as the language she taught. Her cape-dress habit fit smoothly over her corseted torso so that the belt could be snapped at the side with never a wrinkle; no strand of white hair ever escaped the perfect knot beneath her prayer veiling. Yet on occasion, one could detect within the folds of her fleshy cheeks vestiges of earlier dimples, and her eyes still sparkled with merriment.

Miss Kemrer was all about the business of learning Latin, and not a minute should be wasted. Every long mark was important, a clue to the case or conjugation or pronunciation of the words. Her classroom was equipped with large blackboards running the full length of two sides of the room. We were regularly sent to the board to write all seventy-two forms of an indicative verb in its active and passive voices. At first, some of us wrote quickly to get the job done early and rest our weary arms; but after we learned that our reward was to erase and begin a second verb, we wrote more slowly. Miss Kemrer never forgot to assign homework.

My friend Audrey Musser (Murray) and I met regularly in the library to work on our translations as a team and often spent hours trying to tease some sense from our Virgil or Ovid assignments. One day, we decided that we had had enough, that Miss Kemrer's assignments were unreasonable. I am embarrassed to recall how we marched out of the library and down the hall to the office of Dean Ira E. Miller to report that Miss Kemrer's expectations were too high. He welcomed us into his sanctum with a genial smile and listened to our pleas in his kind, attentive way but eventually sent us off with the jovial reminder that "hard work never hurt anyone!"

Miss Kemrer was also my supervising teacher for practice teaching prior to certification. The students were only six or eight years my junior, and I enjoyed laughing with them and making games of some of their assignments. I confess that I let a few diacritical marks slide. At the end, Miss Kemrer gave me a good evaluation, but it did contain the words, "sometimes a little lax!"

Latin was the passport to my first contract as a teacher at Turner Ashby High School in Dayton, Virginia. I was assigned five classes: Latin I and Latin II, and three sections of eighth grade English. It was then that I really learned Latin! My Latin students were the "clever ones" that Sir Winston would have allowed to study the language as an honor, and staying a few paces ahead of them that first year was often a challenge. I remember my *discipuli/ae* with fondness and hope that all the benefits of learning this language are theirs—larger vocabulary and better understanding of many English words—ease in learning other languages, especially modern Romance languages and greater appreciation for the classical foundations of Western civilization.

The highlight for the Latin Club each year was the Roman Banquet when first year students wearing skimpy tunics sewn by their mothers from old sheets were auctioned as slaves to second year students. The "patricians" took delight in ordering their slaves to serve them food and attend to their whims during the banquet and to entertain them afterward with such humiliating relays as pushing grapes across the floor with their noses.

The *mensa* was spread with foods enjoyed by the ancient Romans. It was so customary for eggs to appear in the *gustus* (appetizer) and apples in the *secunda mensa* (dessert) that "from eggs to apples" came to be the Roman way of saying "from start to finish." The Latin students feasted on these and other delicacies including *panis* (bread), sardines, olives, figs, and grape juice wine.

The second meal of the ancient Roman's day was served a little before noon and was the *prandium*, our brunch or lunch. The frittata, a modern day Italian-style omelet, was not known by Julius Caesar, but surely he would have relished it. Fried apples would be an excellent complement.

CHICKEN AND ASPARAGUS FRITTATA

2 tablespoons butter
2 tablespoons onions, finely chopped
6 eggs, lightly beaten
1 cup milk
2 teaspoons ground mustard
1 and ½ cups chopped, cooked chicken
Freshly ground black pepper to taste
8 asparagus spears, canned and drained
¼ cup grated Swiss cheese

Heat the butter in a large pan. Add onions and cook until tender.

Whisk the eggs, milk, and mustard together and pour slowly over the onions. Add chicken and pepper and cook over low heat for fifteen minutes or until frittata is set.

Preheat broiler. Arrange asparagus spears on top of frittata and sprinkle with cheese. Place under hot broiler until the cheese is melted and golden, about two minutes. Serves four.

FRIED APPLES

2 tablespoons butter
6 medium cooking apples, sliced
¼ cup brown sugar
¼ cup orange juice
½ teaspoon cinnamon

Melt butter in small sauce pan. Add apple slices, brown sugar, orange juice and cinnamon. Cover. Bring to rapid boil. Turn heat to low and allow to simmer for twenty minutes. Do not remove lid during cooking. Serves six.

These two "eggs to apples" dishes could be the basics for a wonderful brunch menu—fit for a prime minister! So there you have it, Sir Winston!
Mensa! O Table!

E

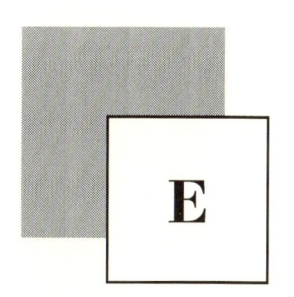

\'ē\ (also e)
n. (pl. es or e's)
the fifth letter of the alphabet

ENGLAND

Recipe: A "Proper" Pot of Tea

Recipe: Cherry Cream Scones

ENGLAND

"Anythingforstarters?"

We looked at each other with puzzled expressions, not because we hadn't decided whether or not to order appetizers but because this greeting didn't register at all with us! We had recently checked through Immigration and gathered our luggage in the Baggage Claim of Heathrow Airport, gone to our hotel for a short nap, and now, hungry, we were seated in a nearby restaurant. The server's question brought us face to face with British intonations and uncustomary word choices, along with foreign restaurant culture. Undoubtedly, a cross-cultural experience lay ahead!

The time was June 1986. Ann, Jill, Jay, and I had come to England for the summer with several purposes. Ann and Jill had just graduated from college and were with us for a two-week family vacation. Then Jay and I were to enroll in a four-week course at the University of London, "British Theater, Literature, and Culture since 1940," a part of Jay's sabbatical program and our orientation to an England we had not seen since 1960. Most importantly, we were on site for the arrival of thirty-six EMC students who would join us in September for the Great Britain Semester in fulfillment of their cross-cultural requirement. Jay was to be their professor, and I was to be his administrative assistant.

The students arrived on schedule, bleary-eyed from their overnight flight. We shepherded them into the waiting coach. (Never call this vehicle a "bus"; that name is reserved for short transports only.) And after stowing their mounds of luggage in the underbelly of the coach, we began the journey to Cambridge. Many slept most of the way. "Studying the backs of their eyelids," our guide commented.

That night, we all slept at the Cambridge YPCA, the following night at the York Youth Hostel, and the night after that in the University of Edinburgh residence halls. Men and women were housed in separate wings, floors, even buildings, and for the entire month of our travels, Jay and I rarely shared a room.

The traditional English breakfast is a substantial pleasure worth arising for! The menu may include any or all of the following: a rasher of bacon, sausages, kippers, gammon, eggs (many varieties), grilled tomatoes, sautéed mushrooms, baked beans, cereals, fried bread, toast, butter and marmalade, juice, coffee, and tea! In Scotland, black pudding was part of the menu, a sausage-like patty made from oatmeal and spices mixed with blood. Our lunches were "on-your-own" in whatever town we happened to stop. We sometimes used this occasion to break up cliques by drawing numbers for lunch partners with the assignment to see which pair could spend the least pounds and pence.

We ate dinner at the place of our lodging, often served with more formality and gleaming cutlery than the students might have preferred. Sometimes the food was new. In the Oxford University dining hall, our "starter" was a lovely platter of whole fried smelt, little beady eyes looking right up at us! Those intent on making the most of new opportunities chose the steak and kidney pie!

Our guide for this tour of Great Britain was Eddie Lerner, an Oxford graduate and a veritable encyclopedia of English literature and history. He essentially taught our "Heritage of Britain" course as we traveled, telling the stories and showing the settings where important events had occurred. "Eddie," our very respected and likeable leader, became the living authority for all things British.

Jay was busy with instruction too. He taught *Macbeth* as we traveled in Scotland. How amazing to look out the window of our coach and see the Birnam Wood we had just met in our reading! Later in the month, Jay taught *Midsummer Night's Dream* before we saw that fanciful performance at the Stratford Theater. Students kept daily journals, reflecting on their experience, and Jay read their writings according to a regular collection schedule.

After we survived the Dominican Convent in Dublin, Ireland, where the furnace was "asunder" and luxuriated in the verdant Bodnant Gardens of Wales, we moved into southern England. There, I taught *The Mayor of Casterbridge*, a novel by Thomas Hardy, as we came into Dorset County, and Jay taught *Murder in the Cathedral* by T. S. Eliot before our visit to Canterbury.

The evening we drove into London for our six-week stay, the coach was strangely quiet. The students were awed but a little anxious by the bigness of the city. We realized that urban life would be a bigger challenge for many than living in this foreign country had been, but we knew they were prepared. They were now familiar with the sounds of British English, the money system, and some customs; and they knew each other. A great bond of camaraderie had developed among the students.

Our "home" was a wing of the Hampstead Heath Youth Hostel located in Golders Green in north London. Jay and I had a room with bunk beds, a table/desk, three chairs, a sink and mirror, but no dresser or closet or clothes hooks. Toilets and showers were less than a block away! Our thirty-six students lived in doubles and triples just beyond the next fire door, so they regularly stopped by our room to talk on their exit or return. Everyone ate a large English breakfast in the dining room each morning before class in the television lounge began at ten o'clock. Once a week while Jay taught, I walked down the street to Barclays Bank and withdrew 1710 pounds, stashed the wad in my big purse, and tried to return nonchalantly in time to dole out the weekly allowances.

Hostel rules required everyone to vacate his or her room from ten to five o'clock that pushed us all into the streets of London every afternoon rain or shine to visit museums, attend free concerts at Saint Martins-in-the-Fields, sketch historic buildings, work on independent studies, or shop in Covent Garden or Oxford Street. The visual and performing arts course involved attendance and brief written reports on concerts, theater productions, films, opera, dance, and art exhibits, consuming many evening hours.

We found a little money left in our discretionary budget before we parted for small group travel on the continent, so we arranged a celebration dinner at Muntaz, an exotic Indian restaurant near Baker Street, where we feasted on tandoori chicken, pilaf, nan, and curries. It was not hard to justify eating this lovely meal in an ethnic restaurant as part of our London cross-cultural experience.

Safely back in the States, we were glad to celebrate Christmas with our biological families, but we keenly missed our cross-cultural family. One evening after everyone was back to campus for second semester, we gathered at a student's home for a reunion. That evening, our students surprised us with a priceless gift—a large photo album full of pictures they had taken en route. (We had not carried a camera in order to have one less encumbrance.) Most important, each student had included a picture of him or herself and a handwritten note of thanks. We were humbled to the point of tears.

In the years that followed, Jay and I led another semester-long cross-cultural trip to Great Britain (1992), two three-week summer courses (1997 and 2001), and a summer jaunt for EMU alumni (1990). Each of these courses was different, but all bore many hallmarks of that first tour.

In 1992, our week in Ireland was memorable for its exposure to life in a conflict-torn country. We entered Northern Ireland and went by coach to Belfast where we visited the Salt Shaker, a coffee shop operated to benefit youth in that Protestant-Catholic torn area of the city, and we had a walking tour of the gang-painted red and blue streets. Later, we visited Corrymeala Reconciliation Center and its heart-shaped worship center and Derry City, site of Bloody Sunday. In Dublin, we heard Joe Leichty, Mennonite Missions worker, tell about his efforts in reconciliation work. Two stays at bed-and-breakfast establishments gave opportunities to experience the warmth of the Irish people in home settings.

Our dear friends Margaret and Herb Swartz joined us for both of the summer three-week programs. Their wit and wisdom enhanced our travels and provided good companionship for Jay and me. On the evening before their early departure in 1997, we managed an invitation to a free rehearsal of *Always,* the love story of Edward and Wallis Simpson, at the Victoria Palace Theatre.

In 1997, the group saw the queen make her way by horse-drawn carriage from Buckingham Palace to Parliament for the opening of the new Labor Party government with Tony Blair as prime minister. The preparations for this short journey required hours of time. We watched city workers wash and vacuum the street, take down light poles, put up fencing to hold back the crowds, and dive in the nearby pools to scan for bombs. Snipers were visible on the palace roof, and bobbies were posted at regular intervals. At last she came, waving her white-gloved hand as the majestic team of horses carried her carriage swiftly past our sight.

After the successful bed-and-breakfast stays in Ireland, we added Home Stays to both of the summer sessions as well as visits to London Mennonite Centre where we enjoyed tea and hospitality while we learned about their program for peace-building in the city.

Occasionally, Jay and I managed to share a romantic day or evening together with no group responsibilities. One Saturday morning in 1997, we began the day by touring the new Globe Theatre then under construction south of the Thames. We were invited to view the rehearsal for a scene from *Winter's Tale* that was set to open the following week.

Later, looking for a place to eat a late lunch, we strolled down the Strand and came upon Simpsons, a name I remembered from our guidebook. Curious and hungry, we went inside the 1828 British establishment and were seated at our damask-covered table in a large wood-paneled dining room. We soon realized that we were in for a pricey meal but decided to call it "our anniversary" (it wasn't) and just enjoy the experience. For starters, we had a salad of Belgium endive and hard rolls. Jay ordered a vegetable flan for his main course, and I had trout with new potatoes and a green vegetable mix. Would we care for dessert? Yes. We ordered the treacle pudding with custard, a rather heavy cake-like serving drowned in caramel syrup and covered with creamy custard—sweet, delicious, and filling. We counted at one point and believed we had each used twelve different pieces of cutlery. The maitre d' wore tails; the servers were all in white jackets. Napkins were monogrammed, and the china and carpets were custom designed with the signature head of a chess piece.

In a splurging mood, we next went to a china shop and bought the last three thimbles of my Brambly Hedge set. That evening, Jay and I topped off our wonderful day by hearing James Galway in a flute concert at the Barbican. As one encore, he played "Danny Boy," my favorite Irish folk melody.

"It was the best of times!"

"It was the worst of times!"

I borrow these words from English novelist, Charles Dickens, to sum up the fact that there were certainly peaks and valleys in our fifteen-year stint as cross-cultural leaders, a career within our other careers! To leave the impression that we had one long holiday in "merrie olde England" would gravely misrepresent our experience.

The task of teaching in these circumstances demanded incredible flexibility. Imagine being the only professor for thirty-six students and offering each of them their total semester's credit. Expect to be on call twenty-four hours a day, every day, for a whole semester. Picture the smoky Goats' Bar at the International Student House as the classroom—no blackboard—and duplicating services too expensive for regular handouts. Add up the endless hours of journal reading and paper grading. Realize that library resources are usually not available for transients, and begin to see the academic challenges a semester abroad can present for a professor.

At times, safety and security were concerns. A journal entry reads, "The IRA continues their bombings. Last night, a taxi was hijacked and taken to 10 Downing Street and was abandoned. A little later, it was blown up by a bomb within." Not infrequently, all trains between the stations named were stopped because of a "suspicious package." Occasionally, there were break-ins and thefts in the youth hostels. We worried about immature students who were out late at night in unfamiliar territory. Students got sick and needed appropriate medical services.

The petty logistical things absorbed huge amounts of patience. Launderettes were few, expensive, dirty, and time consuming. Using the banking system and doling out weekly allowances gave headaches, to say nothing of the faltering exchange rates. Buses or trains ran late and then came two in a row. There were many "dull days," a British expression for rain. Many showers and bathroom facilities must have been installed soon after indoor plumbing was invented. In Scotland, Jay and I remember two showers side by side that were controlled by a single water temperature gauge on the *outside* of the showers. Both bathers needed to agree on the temperature before they took the high steps up into their two shower boxes!

The students were young, usually inexperienced travelers, and they wore their stresses on their sleeves. They brought too much luggage. One coach driver joked that the students "had enough money to go on trips but not enough for house insurance, so they had to bring everything with them!" There were complainers, tattletales, and misfits aboard. Some were hung up on shopping, American food chains, and enough outlets for their curling irons. Others mismanaged their money and incurred debts. The pubs presented temptations. Impressions of a whole country can be colored by the behavior of a traveling group. What did people of other nations think of Americans when our students were greedy at breakfast or took pictures where photography had been forbidden?

Our own personal needs for privacy and concerns about health confronted us. One year, Jay's mother who was suffering from a terminal disease was hospitalized, and we worried that we might be called home.

When things became too bleak and overwhelming, we resorted to one of five potent antidotes for our pain—any of which was more effective than aspirin or tranquilizers! (Indeed, any of these can be enjoyed without an excuse!)

Dillons Bookstore, branded as Waterstone's since 1998, was located in Bloomsbury near the University of London. It was a library for sale but free to any browser who needed to disengage for an hour or so among its impressive array of most books currently in print.

A second escape route was theater. London may hold the title of "Theater Capital of the World" with approximately one hundred theaters in the city and at least fifty in the West End. Each week we bought a copy of *Time Out* and chose our favorites. I wonder how many shows we saw over the years, and I'd be too embarrassed to report the number if I knew!

Regent's Park, an oasis of four hundred acres of green space within the grey concrete pavements of London, gave us a breath of fresh air on many occasions. The serene beauty of Queen Mary's Rose Garden never failed to lift our spirits. The park also housed swans, fountains, promenades, an open-air theater, bandstand, zoo, and tea house.

On Sunday evenings, we frequently attended services at All Souls—Langham Place where we joined hundreds of other Christians in hymn singing and Bible study. One evening, according to my journal, the sermon was based on Exodus, chapter 7. The speaker told us, "It was not that Moses had such great faith in God but that he had faith in a great God." I don't remember why that was significant to me on that particular evening, but it must have been the encouragement I needed.

Finally, if all else failed to restore our stamina, we could always depend on a cup of tea to sustain us. In fact, this marvelous beverage was welcome rain or shine, made in the hot pot in our room or served as part of a fancy cream tea at the Sherlock Holmes Hotel on Baker Street or the Fortnum and Mason in Piccadilly.

Anna, the seventh Duchess of Bedford, is believed to have originated the idea of afternoon tea. She experienced "sinking feelings" every afternoon around four o'clock and asked that a tray of sandwiches and cake and a pot of tea be sent to her boudoir. Later, she began to invite friends to join her and thus began this lovely British national habit.

HOW TO MAKE A "PROPER" POT OF TEA

1. Fill the tea kettle with freshly drawn cold water and put it on to boil.
2. Pour boiling water into the teapot to warm it. Pour out the water before Step 3.
3. Measure a teaspoonful of tea for each cup into a china or glass teapot. Add an extra teaspoonful for the pot.
4. As soon as the kettle comes to a rolling boil, remove it from the heat. Over boiling causes the water to lose oxygen, resulting in a flat brew.
5. Pour boiling water into the teapot and let tea brew three to five minutes.
6. Stir tea gently before pouring it through a tea strainer into the teacups.

An excellent pot of tea deserves bone china cups to drink it from. Jay bought my first Brambly Hedge cup and saucer in the Lake District and gave it to me for my birthday in 1986. I have since collected the complete tea service of this charming "Four Seasons" pattern (Royal Doulton). The artist, Jill Larkin, has created a community of mice who live in Brambly Hedge, "a safe and idyllic spot where old values flourish and self-sufficiency is the order of the day." The bottom of each piece tells a bit of story. On the bottom of the teapot, we read, "They found Mr. Apple in the kitchen drinking mint tea with Mrs. Crustybread."

Mr. Apple and Mrs. Crustybread would have enjoyed my favorite recipe for scones.

CHERRY CREAM SCONES

½ cup dried cherries (or dried cranberries)
1 cup boiling water
3 cups all-purpose flour
3 tablespoons sugar
1 tablespoon baking powder
½ teaspoon salt
½ teaspoon cream of tartar
½ cup butter, room temperature
1 egg, separated
½ cup sour cream
⅔ cup half and half or whole milk
1 teaspoon almond extract (or vanilla)
Additional sugar

Soak cherries in boiling water for ten minutes. Drain and set aside.

In a large mixing bowl, combine the flour, sugar, baking powder, salt, and cream of tartar. Cut in the butter until crumbly. Set aside.

In a small bowl, combine the egg yolk, sour cream, milk, and extract. Add to flour mixture until a soft dough forms. Turn onto a lightly floured surface. Knead gently six to eight times. Knead in cherries.

Separate dough into three balls. Roll each ball into a six-inch circle. Cut into six wedges. Place on lightly greased baking sheet. Beat egg white until foamy and brush tops of rounds. Sprinkle with sugar. Bake at 400 degrees for fifteen minutes or until lightly brown on top. Yield: eighteen scones.

Serve warm with butter and marmalade or whipped cream and fresh strawberries.

F

\'ef\ (also f)
n. (pl. fs or f's)
the sixth letter of the alphabet

FARM FOOD

Recipe: Dandelion Salad with Hot Bacon Dressing

Recipe: Ratatouille

FOREIGN HOSPITALITY

Recipe: Moussaka

FOUNTAIN

Recipe: Ann's Fruit Smoothie

Recipe: Pumpkin Bread

FARM FOOD

What we all don't know about farming could keep the farmers laughing until the cows come home. Except that they are barely making a living, while the rest of us play make-believe about the important part being the grocery store. Animal, Vegetable, Miracle, Barbara Kingsolver, Harper Collins, 2007, p. 12.

Living on a farm was like owning our own supermarket stocked with very fresh, entirely unprocessed foods. Instead of pushing our cart up and down the aisles, we pushed it around the seasons.

Each year, spring finally came, and among the first shoots of new life were the dandelions with their tender notched edges. Just as all kittens and puppies are cute when infants but may grow to be less attractive, so baby dandelions are very pretty in their infancy. Dandelions were one of nature's ways of providing our ancestors with vitamins their winter diet lacked. Mother would take her little aluminum pan and an old paring knife and walk the edges of our garden, looking for enough blades to make a fresh salad with hot bacon dressing. Before long, other greens, such as lettuce and spinach, grew in our garden; and rhubarb, along with its partner, the strawberry, appeared and were made into delicious desserts and jams.

Mother was captain of the summer garden, and the rest of us marched to her orders. We battled our enemy—the weeds—by hoeing and pulling and claimed our victory when an abundance of fresh, beautiful, colorful vegetables appeared. I was never a big fan of garden work; picking green beans made my back ache, and the corn blades stirred up an itchy rash on my arms. For me, the kitchen stage was more enjoyable. Sitting in a circle on the back porch, we shelled peas or strung green beans while we talked and listened to music on our radio.

Canning and freezing were a constant industry throughout the summer. Acid-type foods like tomatoes and peaches were canned with the boiling water bath method. First, enough Mason quart jars were brought from the basement and given a soapy bath. Then we ran a finger around the rim to make sure there were no "nicks" in the glass that would prevent sealing. For peaches, Mother made syrup by heating sugar and water in a saucepan until the sugar dissolved, and we poured boiling water on the new metal lids to soften their rubber ring and make sealing more certain. Since peaches soon darken after they are peeled, we had to work quickly to fill our jars. Sometimes I packed while Mother peeled, stacking the halves into alternating tiers, pit-side down until the jar was full. After the sugar syrup was poured into the jar, one of us ran a table knife between the peaches and the jar to let all the air bubbles escape. Then we carefully wiped the rim, put on the lid, and tightened it with a metal ring. The filled jars were lowered into the canner and covered with hot water where they were allowed to boil for half an hour, jiggling and spitting on their rack. Later, as the jars cooled on the counter, we listened and counted each "ping" as the vacuum seal was formed. Golden peaches, shining in their sugar syrup, are a kitchen art; we thought they were as pretty as any painting as we stood and admired our work.

As summer waned and autumn approached, we planted a row of collards and kale in the garden, froze applesauce, put up a few jars of grape juice, harvested the potatoes, and picked up the black walnuts that had fallen from our tree. Nothing was wasted. The last of the garden vegetables were made into an "end-of-the-garden pickle" that included cauliflower flowerets, tiny green cucumbers, red and green chopped peppers, carrot rings, large lima beans, corn, onions, and celery in pickling brine. Even green tomatoes were picked before the frost to line the window ledges of the laundry room and slowly ripen.

When the winter temperatures became consistently cold enough, we stocked the "meat counter" of our "farm supermarket." Each year, we butchered a beef, two hogs, and numerous chickens, packaged the meat in meal-size servings, and froze it. The carcass of a beef needed to age for about a week in order for the muscles to weaken and become more tender. Daddy used a pulley to hang it from the rafters of our unused garage. Pork did not need this aging time but required so many processes that it took a very long day and several good helpers to complete the task.

Some children stayed home on butchering day, but we were usually sent to school, apparently not considered "essential personnel!" We would come home to find fresh sausage ground into a big dishpan, hams waiting to be sugar-cured, pudding meat in pint jars and its broth mixed into corn meal to be made into ponhoss. Blobs of fat simmered in an iron kettle over an outdoor fire to be rendered into lard. Everything I touched felt greasy. That evening, Mother fried the brains for supper because Daddy claimed to like them, but I turned up my nose and ate only the alternative, a fresh and nicely browned sausage patty.

I was more often involved in the butchering process when we killed a dozen or two broilers and dressed them for the freezer. Daddy or Jim was usually on hand to hold the live chicken by the feet and lay its head on the block for quick execution with a hatchet. It was then doused in a bucket of very hot water to loosen the feathers. Plucking and singeing came next and then the removal of the lower legs and feet. Then the birds were moved to the laundry room where Mother and I completed the task. My first assignment was to hold the chicken by the neck in a pan of warm sudsy water and give it a good bath, removing as many pinfeathers as possible. It was then turned over to Mother and her sharp knife to open the bird and remove the entrails, saving the heart, liver, and gizzard which were considered good in gravy.

We left some birds whole for roasting and cut others into pieces for frying. Finally, each was carefully packaged for the freezer.

The garden and butchering were seasonal, but the laying hens and cows knew no seasons. They produced good eggs and rich milk year round. Sometimes I helped to gather eggs and clean them for market with a little sandpaper brush and helped to wash the buckets and other equipment in the milking parlor.

While Mother's food responsibility centered on food for people, Daddy's realm was food for animals. There were hay fields to mow, grains to plant and harvest, and silos to fill. Occasionally, I drove the tractor as the men picked up hay bales, but I rarely did field work because my father considered it "men's work," and I never protested that assumption! When neighbors helped with threshing or silo filling, I helped Mother cook a big noontime meal for the men who declared that Mother made the best lemon meringue pie in the neighborhood!

Farmers work from sun up to sun down, especially in the summertime. The reward for their long hours at the end of the day is to enjoy the fruits—and vegetables—of their labor at suppertime. Mother always did a good job of bringing the garden to the table. A typical supper menu might have been fried country ham, mashed potatoes or corn on the cob, fresh green beans, sliced cucumbers in a creamy dressing, thick red slices of ripe tomatoes, homemade bread, and sweet iced tea. Fresh sliced peaches from a nearby orchard often provided a simple but delicious dessert.

If I sound nostalgic, it is because I am. It is March, and the "fresh" produce in my refrigerator comes from everywhere. I have a cucumber from Canada, grapes and avocado from Chile, red peppers and parsley from Mexico, and oranges from California. My apples are from Michigan, and the label informs me that they are "coated with food-grade vegetable and/or shellac based wax to maintain freshness!"

In 2012, much of the food on our tables travels a thousand miles or more and comes complete with additives, preservatives, and excess packaging—all of which require energy and generate emissions to create. Just fifty years ago, traditional farmers raised a mixture of crops, and the local food we ate was varied and full of health. In 1963, when I had a cesarean section, my surgeon marveled at how quickly my incision healed. "One thing for sure," he said, "you have had good nutrition."

Now spring comes again and the perennial dandelions are among the first plants ready to brave the changeable temperatures. Jay walks around the border of our lot and finds enough healthy-looking, tender shoots for me to make a salad with hot bacon dressing. We enjoy it once again—just for old times' sake.

DANDELION SALAD WITH HOT BACON DRESSING

4 cups tender dandelion stalks, chopped
2 hard-cooked eggs, sliced
4 slices bacon, fried crisp and crumbled

Dressing

1 tablespoon flour
1 tablespoon sugar
¼ teaspoon salt
Dash of pepper
2 tablespoons vinegar
¾ cup milk

Wash dandelion thoroughly and chop into bite-sized pieces.

Chop bacon and fry until crisp. Remove bacon and reserve two tablespoons drippings.

Mix salt, sugar, and flour; add vinegar and milk and stir until well blended.

Cook sauce in bacon drippings until thickened, stirring constantly.

Pour hot mixture over dandelion and mix lightly.

Garnish with egg slices and crumbled bacon.

Serves three or four persons.

Our small hillside garden plots often disappoint us, so we depend on weekly visits to the wonderful Harrisonburg-Rockingham County Farmers' Market where every local fruit and vegetable is displayed in tempting abundance. At least once each summer, I make sure I buy what I need to make ratatouille, a rich and colorful stew of vegetables. All the vegetables are fresh from Rockingham County; only the recipe originated in the Provençal region of France.

RATATOUILLE

1 large eggplant, unpeeled
Salt

¼ cup olive oil
1 large onion, chopped
2 cloves garlic, minced

2 tablespoons fresh basil, chopped (or 2 teaspoons dried)
1 teaspoon dried oregano
1 bay leaf

2 medium summer squash, cut into one-fourth inch slices
2 red sweet peppers
2 cups tomatoes, peeled, seeded, and chopped
2 tablespoons red wine vinegar
2 teaspoons sugar
Freshly ground black pepper

Cut eggplant into one-half inch cubes. Sprinkle lightly with salt. Place in a colander and let stand for thirty minutes. Wash salt off eggplant and drain well.

In a large saucepan or stockpot, heat the oil. Add onion and garlic and sauté until tender.

Add eggplant, basil, and bay leaf and cook over medium heat until eggplant is tender (about fifteen minutes).

Add summer squash, peppers, tomatoes, and seasonings and simmer until squash and peppers are tender (about fifteen minutes).

Serve over pasta. Sprinkle with chopped fresh parsley, black olives, and freshly grated Parmesan cheese.

Serves 4-6 persons.

FOREIGN HOSPITALITY

To fully appreciate what hospitality can mean, we possibly have to become first a stranger ourselves. Henri J. N. Nouwen, *Reaching Out,* Doubleday and Company Inc., NY 1966, p. 48.

A person is never more a stranger than when visiting a foreign country—foreign foods, foreign currency, foreign sights and smells, foreign language, foreign faces.

My first passport had a green cover and was issued May 1960. The secretary of state fixed his seal and requested "all whom it may concern to permit safely and freely to pass and in case of need to give all lawful aid and protection to the above named citizen of the United States." My several subsequent passport documents, all navy blue in color, have given me the opportunity to again become a "stranger," as Nouwen recommended.

The summer of 1960 began with a day of orientation in New York City, and I had a terrible stomachache! I felt as green as the cover of my passport! It was to be the first airplane ride of my nineteen years, and I would be heading across the Atlantic for eleven weeks of new experiences. I was both excited and fearful; fortunately, the pain subsided when we were airborne and began to enjoy the novelties of KLM 602 (Royal Dutch Airlines).

The 1960 European Educational Tour group flew from Idlewild (now John F. Kennedy), touched down at Prestwick in Scotland long enough to be served a wonderful steak dinner while we waited for our connecting flight to London, and then several days later, we flew to Amsterdam. Six weeks later, three of us flew back to London and then returned to Amsterdam for our departure for the United States, all for $507.60! The cost of the entire trip was $1075, of which $64.03 was later refunded because of savings on land travel—undoubtedly the best bargain of my life!

The three-month summer tour included six weeks of traveling in eight countries (England, Holland, Belgium, France, Switzerland, Italy, Austria, and Germany). We had seats for *Two Gentlemen of Verona* at Stratford Memorial Theatre in England, heard Mahler's music at the Concertgebouw in Amsterdam, delighted in *Rigoletto* at the Opera House in Paris, and attended the Passion Play at Oberammergau in Germany. We wondered at celebrated works of art in the Rijksmuseum, the Louvre, and the Uffizi. We glided through the famous canals of Amsterdam and Venice and cruised on Lake Lucerne and the Rhine River. We were dazzled by Versailles, Windsor Castle, The Hague, and the Palace of the Medici. Cathedrals and sites of historical interest filled our daily schedules.

Italy held special interest for me, having studied Latin for four years. It was textbook come alive to see the Seven Hills of Rome and walk among the ruins of the ancient Forum and Colosseum. In the excavations of Pompeii, we caught glimpses of the ancient Romans' daily lives before the eruption of Mount Vesuvius in AD 79.

The tour, sponsored by the Council of Mennonite Colleges, included many sites of interest to Mennonite students, including Mennonite Central Committee (MCC) centers for peace and material aid work following World War II. We worshiped at the historic Singel Doopsgezinde (Mennonite) Kerk, founded in 1658. In Friesland, the cradle of Mennonitism, we had dinner and spent the night in homes of Dutch Mennonite hosts in the vicinity of Bolsward. I remember the kind hospitality of my hostess, a middle-aged woman whose elderly mother lived with her. She laughed with my friend Audrey and me when we confessed with embarrassment that we had used a large piece of Delft crockery on the floor of the washroom for an unintended purpose because we had not found the separate "water closet" behind an unmarked door further down the hall!

England

When the six weeks of touring had ended the large group dispersed to various work sites for five weeks, many to aid in rebuilding areas destroyed by the war. Jay and I and Mary Burkholder from Canada returned to London to teach children in two separate Summer Bible Schools. Our home, away from home, was the London Mennonite Centre, 14 Shepherds Hill, Highgate, an outstanding place of hospitality.

The London Mennonite Centre, a large fourteen-room, four-story residence in North London, served multiple purposes. It was a place of worship, a student hostel, a guest house for travelers, and an information center. Quintus and Miriam Leatherman were the Mennonite Board of Missions host couple during our stay. We were welcomed as guests but assigned tasks like family members. We peeled potatoes, helped in the garden, and vacuumed the carpets in exchange for a seat at Mrs. Leatherman's table and a cot with clean sheets in one of the large upstairs bedrooms.

Each morning, Mary, Jay, and I rode London's red double-decker buses to either Free Gospel Hall at 39 Grafton Terrace or the Finsbury Mission, Goswell Road, to assist John and Eileen Coffman with one of the two Bible Schools. My poor little Cockney, first and second graders, had trouble understanding my English, and I theirs! We were usually exhausted when the morning was finally over. At that point, John always brought Eileen a steaming cup of tea. How good it looked, we thought, as we viewed his loving gesture with envy!

Our other "religious duties" included Sunday morning and evening services at the London Mennonite Center, midweek meetings, ladies' teas, and occasional visits to the home for old-age pensioners. Jay often sang in quartets, and I read scripture or poured tea. Still, we managed to pack in many visits to London's celebrated sights.

The European Educational Tour of Summer 1960 significantly broadened my college education, and on a personal level, it moved me in the direction of greater autonomy as an adult.

Middle East and the Mediterranean

Much of western people's understanding of the expectations of gracious hospitality is traceable to the Middle East and Mediterranean world. Even the word "hospitality," derived from the Latin *hospes,* is variously translated as "guest, visitor, host, and stranger."

The myth of Baucis and Philemon illustrates the importance of hospitality in the classical world. In this story, Jupiter and Mercury visited the land of Phrygia disguised as peasants. All the residents of the land turned them away until they came to the simple dwelling of the elderly couple, Baucis and Philemon, who invited them inside and treated them with the best they had. When the couple realized that their wine bowl always remained full no matter how much was served, they knew that their guests were actually gods. As a reward for their hospitality, the gods saved them from the flood that soon destroyed their inhospitable neighbors and granted them their wish of never having to live alone. They became oak and linden trees growing together from one trunk.

The biblical writer of Hebrews (13:2) instructed his readers "not to forget to entertain strangers, for by so doing, some people have entertained angels without knowing it."

When more than seventy-five people signed up to travel with EMC President Myron Augsburger on the Third Bible Lands Pilgrimage in 1978, arranged by Travel Counsellors of Harrisonburg, President Augsburger invited professors Herb Swartz and Jay Landis and their spouses to join the tour as assistants. The seventeen-day tour included a four-day cruise to the Greek Isles and Turkey departing from Athens.

We landed in Amman, Jordan, late at night and were pounced on by porters vying for the privilege of carrying our luggage for a small tip. A short time later, we arrived at our hotel, and although we were bedraggled from short nights and time zone changes and wanted only a bed, we must first be served a fine meal. I remember the first course—delicious hot cream of tomato soup, bread, and butter.

After a short night and an early breakfast, we were on our way to Petra, the Red Rose City and its temples carved from multicolored stones, an important caravan center during the first century. We rode horses down the narrow cliff to the rediscovered city. My horse was led by a Bedouin man with limited

English who politely engaged me in conversation and proudly told me that he had "two madams," clearly a measure of his status.

Several days later, Samir Abu Iznaid's father met us unexpectedly at our hotel in Jerusalem. Samir had been an international student from Dura-Hebron, Palestine, at EMC that year, and when his father learned that leaders from his son's college in the States were visiting, he came to greet us and bring us gifts. One of my gifts was a long black dress of polished cotton with flowing sleeves and panels of exquisite hand-embroidered flowers in pinks and reds and purples. The dress was old, even repaired under the arms. I imagine it belonged to one of his wives, possibly a family heirloom, judging from the beauty of the handwork and the fact that it had been altered at the waistline to accommodate a shorter wearer. Samir's father walked with a crutch and a cane and appeared much less prosperous than the travelers in our group. I felt very humbled by his generous hospitality, giving a personal item of family worth to a person he didn't know. I have kept the dress these thirty plus years, wearing it only once and wondering how to bless the hands that embroidered those beautiful flowers.

We visited Israel and Jerusalem during Easter season, an especially meaningful time to see the geography of Jesus's life on earth. Early on Easter Sunday, we attended the sunrise service at the Garden Tomb. During the same day, we visited the Mount of Olives, the Garden of Gethsemane where the ancient olive trees are believed to be the same that observed Jesus in prayer, the Wailing Wall, and the unspeakably beautiful Dome of the Rock. That afternoon, Herb and Margaret Swartz, who had been Mennonite Central Committee workers in Hebron previously, took Jay and me to the Jerusalem Oriental Restaurant where Arabic food was served in a setting decorated as the interior of a Bedouin sheik's tent. We sat on low couches around a brass tray table and savored our salad, hummus, and Arabic breads followed by shish kabobs and tea.

On day nine of the journey, we left behind the names familiar to readers of the Old Testament and the Gospels and flew to Athens to see the remnants of places named in the Epistles of the New Testament. From the magnificent Acropolis, we viewed Mars Hill. In Epidaurus, the group sang "Oh, God, Our Help in Ages Past" in the remains of the sixteen-thousand-seat amphitheater still with perfect acoustics; and in ancient Corinth, we visited the temple of Apollo and the Roman ruins where Saint Paul lived for more than a year of his life.

The four-day cruise in the Aegean Sea on the MTS Galaxy took us first to Mykonos, a white-washed island catering to tourists. Here I bought my favorite ring, an 18-carat gold Gordian knot which I have worn almost constantly ever since. Other ports of call brought us to Ephesus, Patmos, Rhodes, Crete and the Palace of Knossos, Santorini, and back again to Athens. Sometimes the sea was rough and when we staggered from side to side as we made our way to the dining room on a lower deck we were reminded of Saint Paul's shipwrecks.

If the 1960 trip was one of the "best bargains" of my life, the 1978 trip was certainly one of the best gifts of my life. The Middle East, a non-Western culture, took me farthest from home. It helped me realize that Jesus, whom I tend to think of in the context of my own culture, transcends all cultures—all time—and the barriers that easily divided people then and do today.

Italy

Much of our travel abroad during the fifteen-year period from 1986 to 2001 was in association with cross-cultural and alumni office programs at Eastern Mennonite University. On one of the semester trips, we decided to spend our week of vacation in Italy. With our *Berlitz* dictionary in hand, but no competence in the Italian language, we boarded a plane at Gatwick Airport outside London and flew to Pisa. There we found the *treno stazione* and bought *biglietto*s for Florence.

It was late in the afternoon, and the train was crowded. We found seats in a cubicle with two seats facing ours. The swarthy man across from us by the window propped his elbow on the sill and watched the passing landscape while we rode together into the darkening evening. As we neared the city, he turned his attention to us and inquired where we were staying. We had pre-booked a hotel but had no idea where it was located, so we asked him if he knew the place. When we arrived in Florence, he picked up my bag and motioned for us to follow him across the stone pavement and down a dark street. As we scurried along, I wondered at my naïve trust; but eventually, we came to the lighted sign of our hotel. He set my bag on the step, brushed away our thanks, and disappeared into the night. We were certainly the strangers in this story, and we believed him to be the angel!

Later in the week, Jay proposed that we travel to Ravenna, the historic city in northern Italy famous for its early Christian architecture and beautiful mosaics. Once again, we purchased *biglietto*s and found ourselves viewing the scenery as we clacked along. Suddenly the train came to a stop in the middle of nowhere. People around us nonchalantly picked up their parcels and began to exit. Where were they going? Why had we stopped? Like sheep, we rolled our suitcases off the train and also boarded the waiting bus. When the bus was jammed full of people, we took off to somewhere. An aging lady in scarf and shawl studied me seriously and pitied my bewilderment. Somehow, she communicated that we were to follow her, and she would take care of us. Later, the bus stopped abruptly, and we followed her off and into a different waiting train. Eventually, we rolled into Ravenna, never knowing how we got there!

These two nameless "angels" represent countless nameless people whose cordiality has aided our journeys and assured us that many people of all nationalities are not strangers, only friends whose languages we cannot speak.

England and Ireland

The bed-and-breakfast hospitality industry in England and Ireland is big business, attractive to the foreign traveler because it offers a closer look, even *names* of real people who live in real homes. We spent the night in quite a few B and Bs during these fifteen years; all showed respect for us as guests and met our needs. Several names remain along with a memory of their exceptional hospitality.

Sarah and Clive Snell, their three children—Joe, Connie, and Victoria—along with one cat, one ferret, one hundred Friesian dairy cows, and many pigs and piglets lived on a farm near Salisbury, England. Sarah was a good cook whose secret was the use of fresh vegetables grown on the family farm. During our after dinner conversation, we learned that they were active in several farmers' organizations and community government. Family life held high priority. When we retired to our bedroom in the one-hundred-year-old farmhouse, we found the windows wide open, curtains flapping in the fifty-degree breeze. Next morning, we left the windows closed; but when we returned that afternoon, they were open, and the room was "fresh" once again! I liked Sarah and her philosophy of food and nutritious cooking methods.

In 1992, our group arrived in Belfast, Ireland, and began our visit with a stop at the Salt Shaker, a little coffee shop with services for youth, elderly, and handicapped persons in a war-torn neighborhood. Derek McCorkel, the director, took us for a walk through the Catholic and Protestant areas where we saw the wall painting, the boarded up houses, the dirty streets, and the red, blue, and white gutters in the Protestant areas. Later in Derry City, we heard more about Bloody Sunday and other historic incidents. Police and military personnel were everywhere. That evening, we drove across the border and jostled over the rough roads of the Republic of Ireland to the town of Sligo.

Tess and Sean Haughey were the owners of "Rathnashee," Fort of the Fairies, named because an ancient fairy ring was located nearby. Tess and Sean, a couple about our age, welcomed us and several of our students as though we were members of their own family, and we took our places at their table for the best meal of "comfort food" I have ever eaten. My journal records two meats—turkey and gammon, four vegetables—potatoes, parsnips, cabbage, and carrots—preceded by a crusty brown bread and delicious soup and followed by apple tort with custard and cream—all warm, tart, sweet, and spicy. Finally, we were served tea or coffee, cheese and crackers.

Comfort food was what we craved after two days of focusing on wars and conflicts, but more comforting than the food was the reconciling perspective of people who lived with optimism and believed that peace was obtainable for Ireland. Sean collected antiquarian books about Irish history and worked for the forestry service. Tess operated Town and Country Homes, the bed-and-breakfast organization in Sligo. We were privileged to be assigned to her own home; I am certain she and Sean were the best in the business!

Maritime Provinces

The early August 2002 tour to Nova Scotia, Prince Edward Island, and New Brunswick, arranged by TourMagination, began in Halifax and continued for eleven lovely days of scenic beauty on the Cabot Trail, whale watching to Peggy's Cove, lobster dinners, and Bay of Fundy tides. On my birthday, August 7, we were in Charlottetown where we saw the thoroughly entertaining *Anne of Green Gables* musical at the Confederation Center of the Arts.

We invited ourselves to two places, or rather our tour leader did, but the hospitality was just as warm, and it defined the difference between "tourist" and "guest." On Saturday, and again on Sunday, we met some of our Anabaptist brothers and sisters who live in the Maritime Provinces.

After an early Saturday morning bus ride, we arrived at the Petitcodiac Mennonite Church in New Brunswick. Members of the church invited us in to a breakfast feast of fresh fruit, muffins, pancakes, ham, and coffee. The pastor, Werner DeJong, led a thoughtful meditation about work and rest, comparing the intertidal zone sea life to our own water-in, water-out rhythms. Afterward, he told us about the Petitcodiac church and its transformation from liquor store to house of worship—spirits to Spirit! The membership of forty to fifty individuals are some of the few Anabaptists living in the Maritime Provinces and are mostly professionals who want to stay in contact with other members of their faith.

On Sunday morning, our denominational kinship was not as close, perhaps more like cousins than brothers and sisters. After breakfast in Truro, we traveled over hill, dale, and dusty roads to the Northfield Kleine Gemeinde Church. The Kleine Gemeinde group began in Russia and immigrated to North America in 1874 in an attempt to provide farming opportunities for landless members and avoid political involvement. Later, some branches of the Kleine Gemeinde changed their name to Evangelical Mennonite Conference and expanded to various mission posts beyond Manitoba. The Kleine Gemeinde we visited retained that name, immigrated to Belize and later back to Canada. They were a prosperous group in Belize and became the targets of persecution and thievery. Six families left Belize in 1983 and moved to Nova Scotia where they grew to number approximately fifty family units.

We received a warm *Willkommen* from the leader who explained that the men and women should sit on opposite sides of the white-framed church building. We were given a half-page bulletin written entirely in German that contained several scripture verses, names of leaders, and prayer requests for *Sonntag, der 11.*

The women all wore a dark solid-colored dress with a small black kerchief. The men wore black pants and white shirts with no coat or tie. Most of the younger women held a baby and little children were everywhere, sitting patiently beside their mothers. Although German was certainly the preferred language, attempts were made to include their visitors by using English in some songs, prayers, and parts of the sermon. We learned from the preacher's son that his father had never preached in English before and had worked hard all week on his sermon, which was on the theme of trust.

The hospitality extended to dinner invitations in their homes. Jay and I were invited to the home of the preacher and his wife, Klaas and Maria Penner. Maria served a pot roast, garden lettuce, Jello, and ice cream in her simple home. Everything in the house was basic with no artifacts, artistic use of color, or decorative touches to please the eye. I helped her wash the dishes at the small kitchen sink before Klaas took us all on a drive in the dusty station wagon through the community, showing us more of the church where they also operate their own school and have a baling center from which they ship clothing to the Ukraine.

France

It all began the spring of 2007 when friends Carroll and Nancy Yoder were invited to manage the Mennonite Center in Paris while the director was on furlough for the summer and said, "Why don't you come over for a visit?" Then Jay retired after fifty years of teaching, and French professor Chantal Logan said, "Come over to France, and I'll cook you a French dinner!" Ray and Vi Horst were excited about going too, so the trip to France, Summer 2007, was born.

The four of us flew to Lyon, but the checked luggage for Ray, Jay, and me did not! (Wisely Vi packed light and carried hers with her.) Cherishing the hope that it would catch up with us, we picked up our rental car, a VW Passat with stick shift and diesel engine, and motored to Orange, a beautiful city that glowed golden in the evening street lights. After a late *cornet m de glace*, we found our beds for several hours of badly needed sleep.

With no luggage on the scene and hope wavering, we found the large "Auchan" which we were promised "had everything" and purchased a change of clothing and essentials such as deodorant and hair spray. The hand lotion I thought I bought turned out to be liquid soap! (The only one among us with a little French language facility was Ray.) To conclude this part of the story, I sadly report that we never saw our luggage again until it landed on our doorstep some three weeks after we were home. To be a stranger in a foreign country is disconcerting enough, but to be a stranger with no clothing except what is on your back and on your way to Paris, the fashion capital of the world, is surely the stuff of nightmares!

In Le Puy-en-Valay, we were greeted according to the French custom with three kisses (cheek to cheek and kiss the air) by our hosts Chantal and Mark Logan. The Logans own a one-hundred-and-fifty-year-old family home with wooden shutters, lace curtains, and flower boxes in the windows. We soon felt at home—transformed as we crossed the threshold from traveling strangers into welcome house guests.

Chantal fulfilled her promise, prepared, and served an elegant dinner in numerous courses that we savored as we conversed together for several hours. Even the menu makes my mouth water!

> Melon
> Terrine de poisson (a cold fish pate, served with bread)
> Magret de canard a la verveine (filet of duck breast)
> Lentilles du Puy (a lentil specialty of the region)
> Salad
> Fromage (eight varieties of cheese)
> Fruite (fresh cherries, apricots, and peaches)
> Espresso
> Madelines
> Cotes de Provence (rose wine)

When we said goodbye the next morning, Mark loaned Jay a light jacket and a carry-on suitcase and joked that we should come again, with or without luggage!

Our journey took us on through the Loire Valley, splendid even in the rain, to Villandry, the "most beautiful gardens in France" then to the cathedral towns of Tours, Orleans, and Chartres (a must-see for Jay) where we left our car and boarded a train for Paris.

As the friendly faces of Carroll and Nancy emerged from the hurrying crowd at the train station, we knew we were "home" again. They helped us travel via our new Metro cards to the Mennonite Center where Nancy soon served a delicious lunch of pate and olives and a casserole of Belgium endive and ham topped with a cheese sauce.

In the several days that followed, they showed us the beauty of Paris—the Seine, Luxembourg and Tuileries Gardens, Musee D'Orsay, Latin Quarter, Pompidou Center, Eiffel Tower, Sainte Chappelle, Arc de Triomphe, Mont Martre, and the Champs-Elysees. We heard an organ concert at Notre Dame Cathedrale and a concert of three boys' choirs at the Church of Saint Eustache.

Most memorable, however, were the occasions of eating and visiting together. Relaxing breakfasts of cereal, fruit, cheese, and bread stretched into the midmorning. A visit to the fantastic Saturday market to see the stalls of colorful fruits and vegetables, fish, cheeses, olives, breads, and anything-you-want resulted in lunch on the benches of a school play yard. On the evening before our departure, Carroll and Nancy invited us to the Yoder Creperie where we began with fresh cantaloupe, followed by a bolognaise bake (crepes with a creamy meat, cheese, and tomato sauce) and a salad and concluded with a dessert of crepes spread with chocolate and hazelnuts, tea, or coffee.

The French have a reputation for fine food and wine, which I'm perfectly willing to applaud, especially if it is eaten in the company of fine friends. Food is basic to sustain the life of our physical bodies as God designed in our creation. However, I'm certain his plan had a larger dimension as well that the spirit also should be nourished as we eat in company with others. Logans and Yoders brought excellent food into that finer feast.

Russia

In September 2008, we stepped aboard the MS Russ, our riverboat-cruise ship, and were greeted by Russian folk music from accordion and guitar played by men in red jackets and by bread and salt *(khleb da sol)* offered to us by young women in Slavic costumes. The tradition of offering bread and salt to guests spawned the Russian word for hospitality *(khlebosolny)*, bread being the most respected food and salt associated with long friendship. Later in the week, we went to a Russian Tea Ceremony where the tea was served from a large samovar, also a symbol of hospitality.

The ship's crew was Russian, as was our guide, Natalya. She was a spunky, short woman in her sixties and capable of being a little brusque at times. In general, she made her opinions quite palatable by injecting a droll sense of humor and a touch of cynicism into her lectures. She had been a professor of sixteenth century history and had a wealth of knowledge and life experience during several political periods. "All people and every place is wonderful," she said. "It is just our rulers who make life hard for us!"

Our meals were usually eaten on the ship in the Volga Restaurant. The breakfast buffet catered to everyone's whim. Lunch and dinner were served by waiters who took our orders the previous day. The same dining room surprised us each day as we entered and found every table decked in a new color of cloth and fresh flowers. Evening meals were often theme-based—a birthday celebration, a pirate's banquet, or the captain's dinner. Presentation was everything! Who would have guessed there were so many ways to present a cucumber in fanciful design! Presentation is an important aspect of hospitality. The extra touch and thoughtful gesture communicate to guests that they are worth the effort.

One meal of our Russian trip was different from the rest. It was served to our group of forty in a small assembly room in the First Baptist Church in Moscow by ladies wearing large bibbed aprons with their hair tied back by scarves, babushka-style.

At one time, there were about one hundred thousand Mennonites in Russia, many of whom had emigrated there from Germany. After 1945, hundreds of people of German descent were rounded up by the Red Army and forcibly repatriated to Siberia. As they were able, many of the Mennonites left Russia and moved to Canada and the United States so that today, there are only about two thousand Mennonites left in Russia, most living in western Siberia. The few who remain in Moscow have joined the First Baptist Church that, for a long time, was the only Protestant church in the city.

The interior of the building is beautiful with a large pipe organ and seating for one thousand two hundred people. The church has a large membership and five choirs. We sat in the balcony to hear a deacon and a woman who had once worked for Mennonite Central Committee tell us about the growth of the Protestant faith in Russia in recent years.

Our simple lunch began with borscht and bread. The main course was roasted chicken, mashed potatoes, cucumber, and tomato slices. We were served a fruit punch beverage—no dessert.

The language barrier prohibited most communication with our hosts, but the spirit of Christian fellowship prevailed. We sang several hymns for them, and they prayed with us when we arrived and when we left.

Some say that the offering of bread and salt originated as a Christian tradition. Bread was considered a gift from God, and the bread maker made the sign of the cross in the dough many times as it was kneaded. Often, a cross was cut into the top of the loaf before it was baked. The salt, considered a costly treasure, was blessed by the church on Epiphany and dropped into the mouth of one being baptized to preserve the soul.

I understand what Henri Nouwen meant when he said we must first become a stranger ourselves in order to appreciate the meaning of hospitality. In turn, he would understand what I mean when I say that there is a time when we are "strangers no more but part of one humanity." Many times, that happens around the table.

> There is a love that binds the world together,
> A love that seeks the last, the lost, the least.
> One day, that love will bring us all together in Christ
> From South and North, from West and East.
>
> For we are strangers no more, but members of one family;
> Strangers no more, but part of one humanity;
> Strangers no more, we're neighbors to each other now;
> Strangers no more, we're sisters and we're brothers now.

Text: Kenneth I. Morse, 1979, *Hymnal: A Worship Book,* Mennonite Publishing House, Scottdale, PA, 1992

Many recipes and many hours of preparation lie behind the foods we enjoy as travelers. Often, they are once-in-a-lifetime experiences. We cannot duplicate the taste of fried fish eaten in a picnic lunch on a hillside above the Sea of Galilee. Other times, we can approximate the pleasure of that first time experience. It was in a resort-type restaurant somewhere between Athens and Corinth in Greece that I first tasted Moussaka. The flavors surprised and delighted me, so I looked for a recipe and found that there are many. This recipe is much like the dish I remember, but it is rich, and it is large, so do invite some "strangers" to eat it with you!

MOUSSAKA

Ingredients

3 medium eggplants, partially peeled and cut into one-half-inch thick slices
¼ cup olive oil

Meat Sauce
1 tablespoon butter
1 pound lean ground beef
Salt and ground black pepper to taste
1 large onion chopped
1 clove garlic, minced
½ teaspoon ground cinnamon
¼ teaspoon ground nutmeg
½ teaspoon crushed dried oregano
2 tablespoons dried parsley

1 (8 ounce) can tomato sauce
½ cup red wine
1 egg beaten

Béchamel Sauce
4 cups low-fat milk
½ cup butter
6 tablespoons all-purpose flour
Salt and ground white pepper to taste

1 and ½ cup freshly grated Parmesan cheese
¼ teaspoon ground nutmeg

Directions

1. Sprinkle eggplant lightly with salt; stand in colander for an hour to draw out the moisture. Rinse in cold water; drain well. Squeeze out excess moisture with paper towels. Then in a hot skillet, heat the olive oil and fry the eggplant a few slices at a time until tender and golden; remove from pan and drain on paper towels.
2. In a large skillet over medium heat, melt the butter and add the ground beef, salt and pepper, onions, and garlic. When the beef is browned, sprinkle in the cinnamon, nutmeg, oregano, and parsley. Add the tomato sauce and wine. Mix well and simmer for twenty minutes. Allow to cool and then stir in beaten egg.
3. To make the béchamel sauce, begin by scalding the milk in a saucepan. Melt the butter in a large saucepan over medium heat. Whisk in flour until smooth. Lower heat; gradually pour in the hot milk, whisking constantly until it thickens. Season with salt and white pepper.
4. Arrange a layer of eggplant in a greased nine-by-thirteen-inch baking dish. Cover eggplant with all of the meat mixture, and then sprinkle one half cup of Parmesan cheese over the meat. Cover with remaining eggplant, and sprinkle another one half cup of cheese on top. Pour the béchamel sauce over the top, and sprinkle with the nutmeg. Sprinkle with the remaining cheese.
5. Bake for one hour at 350 degree. Serves eight.

FOUNTAIN

There is a fountain in the Historic Quad of Thomas University in southwestern Georgia bearing a bronze plaque with the names of Dr. Jay B. and Mrs. Peggy H. Landis.

It happened this way.

In summer 1994, our daughter Ann moved to Tallahassee, Florida, to begin her PhD program in Humanities at Florida State University. Ann's next four years were filled with intense study, teaching, and dissertation writing. Occasionally, she found time to relax and enjoy the unique culture of Florida's panhandle. When we could, Jay and I visited, often in March when we needed a warm midterm break. Then our "tour guide," Ann, led us to excellent restaurants with seafood straight from the Gulf, strolled with us among the azaleas of Maclay Gardens State Park, and took us for scenic drives on live oak-lined roads overhung with Spanish moss canopies.

In her fourth year, Ann took an adjunct teaching assignment at Thomas University, a short drive across the Florida state line into southwestern Georgia. Thomas University is a four-year accredited private university that awards associate, bachelor, and master's degrees to a student body of one thousand students.

The main building and grounds were originally part of Birdwood Plantation, once owned by Ambassador W. Cameron Forbes. In 1950, the Primitive Baptist Church chartered a junior college on the site that became nonsectarian and independent by 1979 and grew by 2000 to be Thomas University. It is mostly a commuter campus where a large number of adult students complete or advance their professional careers.

Thomas University is located in Thomasville, a small town of Southern grace and charm that maintains over seven thousand rose bushes and calls itself the City of Roses. During the Victorian Era, Thomasville was known as the Winter Resort of the South. Today, the sprawling plantations, historic museums, and grand mansions are reminiscent of that era.

Ann was employed by Thomas University in 1998 as a full-time assistant professor of English. Since then, she has moved administratively from division chair to associate dean, to dean of arts and sciences, to vice president for academic affairs. In 2010, she was also named provost.

Along the way, Susan Otto, originally from Wisconsin, was appointed to the nursing faculty at Thomas. When she completed her PhD in nursing in 2009, she became the division chair of nursing.

Ann and Sue became good friends and eventually joined households in a comfortable home in Tallahassee. They have become partners in many ways, sharing their commitment to the education of college students, their love of dogs (specifically Bunchie and Casey), and their enjoyment of gardening, sports, and travel. Ann and Sue were each born a twin—one explanation for the name of their boat, Two-of-a-Kind.

When Thomas University undertook a five-million-dollar campus improvement project in 2009, plans called for a fountain in the center of the Historic Quad with sidewalks leading away like spokes to older campus buildings. When we visited Ann and Sue in October 2000, there was no hint of a fountain, only yellow tape and mud, unfinished sidewalks, and the little Primitive Baptist chapel aloft on steel girders waiting to be moved to its new location.

In June 2010, Ann and Sue visited us. One evening, they showed us pictures of recent trips—Sue to Nicaragua with a group of nursing students, and Ann, Sue, and another colleague to China to explore international nursing education programs.

"Oh, one more thing," they said as we wrapped up the China trip. "Here are some pictures of our new campus!"

We were delighted with the new green grass, spick-and-span little chapel, and inviting sidewalks that led to a pretty wrought iron central fountain. Imagine our surprise when they handed us a folder with a picture of a brass plaque bearing the words

The Landis Fountain
Dedicated in the Year 2010
In Honor of
Dr. Jay B. and Peggy H. Landis
for their lifelong commitment to
teaching excellence and the liberal arts
Donated by Dr. Ann Landis and Dr. Susan Otto.

In October, Dr. Gary Bonvillian, president, requested "the honor of our presence for the dedication ceremony of the Landis Fountain." Somehow, we recovered sufficiently from a severe attack of humility and unworthiness and made plans to attend the dedication ceremony.

The Georgia sun was warm and bright that day and made the droplets from the fountain's spray shine like little diamonds. We went first to Ann's dark-paneled office in the Forbes Building to pin on a corsage and boutonnière of red roses and then took our places on two of the white folding chairs on the lawn. Dr. Karl Barton from the music department played a "Brandenburg Concerto" by J. S. Bach on his flute before the vice president of advancement welcomed the guests. A member of the board of trustees thanked Ann and Sue, the donors, and made inspirational comments about the symbolism of the fountain and its waters.

Ann spoke next, a gracious tribute to us that began, "Sue and I want to dedicate our gift of the fountain to my parents because of two gifts they have shared not only with us but with many others over the years: commitment to teaching excellence and a love and appreciation of the liberal arts." She told about our careers in teaching and administration, warming our hearts, not only by her words but by her radiance and strong communication skills. Never mind about our work—it was Ann herself that made us proud!"

After Ann and Sue unveiled the plaque, Dr. Bonvillian concluded the program and invited everyone to have refreshments on the new plaza. We met many of Ann and Sue's colleagues who assured us of their love and respect for Ann and Sue and their leadership.

So our names are on the fountain of a Georgia university whose name we have only known for about a dozen years, a little like two fish out of the pool of water, but we are honored to be named inasmuch as the name may remind future students of Thomas University's academic vice president and provost.

As always, our five-day visit with Ann and Sue was pleasant and relaxing. One morning, we lounged on chairs by their backyard pool while we watched Bunchie and Casey sniff out mysterious intruders in the pine needles and chase phantom squirrels back into their branches. A cool glass of Ann's fruit smoothie, along with a slice of the pumpkin bread I had brought from Virginia, made a delicious conclusion to our breakfast as we discussed "Winter's Bone," the movie we had seen the night before.

ANN'S FRUIT SMOOTHIE

1 and ½ cups vanilla yogurt
2 or 3 medium bananas, ripened
1 cup fresh sliced strawberries
1 cup fresh blueberries
¼ cup milk
1 tablespoon honey
2 tablespoons cold-milled golden flax seed
10 ice cubes

Place all ingredients in a blender. Process on high for one to two minutes until smooth.

Serve immediately. Serves two.

PUMPKIN BREAD

2 and ½ cups sugar
1 cup vegetable oil
4 eggs, lightly beaten
1 can (15 ounces) pumpkin
2 and ½ cups unbleached all-purpose flour
1 cup white whole wheat flour
1 teaspoon baking soda
½ teaspoon baking powder
½ teaspoon salt
1 teaspoon cinnamon
1 teaspoon nutmeg
¼ teaspoon cloves
¼ teaspoon allspice

½ cup water

½ cup chopped golden raisins (optional)
½ cup chopped walnuts (optional)

In a large bowl, mix sugar, oil, and eggs. Add pumpkin and mix well.

Combine flours, baking soda, baking powder, salt, and spices.

Add dry ingredients to the pumpkin mixture alternately with water beating well after each addition.

Mix in raisins and walnuts by hand.

Pour into two greased nine-inch-by-five-inch-by-three-inch loaf pans. Bake at 350 degree for sixty minutes or until a toothpick comes out clean. Cool for ten minutes on wire rack before removing from pans. Cool completely before slicing.

Makes two loaves.

G

\\'jē\\ (also g)
n. (pl. gs or g's)
the seventh letter of the alphabet

GRANDCHILDREN

Recipe: Baked Salmon Filets Dijon

Recipe: Blueberry-Stuffed French Toast

Recipe: Poppy Seed Salad Dressing

Recipe: Swiss Cashew Tossed Salad

Recipe: Mandarin Strawberry Salad

GRANDPARENTS HEATWOLE

Recipe: Sugar-Cured Country Ham

GRANDPARENTS SUTER

Recipe: Skillet-Fried Chicken

Recipe: Oven-Fried Chicken

GRANDCHILDEN

I turned sixty, and Jay planned a birthday dinner celebration for our family with all four generations present, from Grandma Dot to tiny Baby Tim. Mother's best-ever fresh coconut cake, Ann's parmesan chicken, and Jill's mandarin salad were good parts of the menu. Becky, still five for another week, and Nate, soon-to-be three, came with mischief in their eyes and a plate of sixty circus peanuts—those creamy orange marshmallow candies shaped like nuts. It was a joke for an aging grandmother who should no longer like such a wacky treat but did and even more so when given by her grandchildren!

It is doubtful that Becky and Nate remember this occasion since it would not be considered a significant event, like the birth of a sibling. Psychologists call the relative scarcity of memories held by young children before the age of five years "childhood amnesia," a phenomenon that may result from lack of neurological development, incomplete language development, or differences in the perspective from which children and adults experience the world. Whatever the cause, most adults cannot access many memories from early childhood or cannot distinguish between the actual memory of an event and the knowledge of an event based on pictures or the stories of someone else.

In this case, the "stories of someone else" are mine—selected memories from their earliest years told from a grandma's perspective.

In the summer of 1993, we waited and waited, almost prisoners in our own home lest we miss the call, until Craig's voice finally informed us that Rebecca Karis had arrived on August 16. We hurried to pack the car and headed to Meridian, Mississippi, arriving in time for our first sight of tiny Becky, dark-haired and fast asleep in her hospital bassinette. When her hair turned blond with soft curls about two years later, our waiter called her "seriously beautiful" and summoned fellow waiters to come and have a look at his darling little customer.

In October 1996, the call came from North Port, Florida, announcing the birth of Nathaniel Jay. This time, we took a plane to the Sarasota-Bradenton Airport, secured our rental car, and rushed to the hospital to see the cutest little "pumpkin" ever born on Halloween Day!

Timothy Elijah was born in the same Florida hospital on May 18, 1999, and Craig woke us with the good news about one o'clock in the morning. We could hear Timmy's energetic crying in the background. After the sun was up, Jill called again to say that he was "so pretty with pink skin, a little round face, and dark hair," much like Becky and Nate's had been. This time, we had to wait several days before going, so that Jay could finish giving second semester exams.

By now, Becky was completing a happy year in kindergarten, and Nate was ready to assume big brother authority. The Sniders were selling their house and planning a move to Virginia in July 1999. One morning, Jay and I helped to get the house ready for a real estate agent's visit before taking Nate with us on some errands. Soon after the three of us had sat down at a table in McDonalds with tall glasses of cold orange juice, a little hellion, a year or two older than Nate, arrived with his mother and ran berserk around the restaurant, finally stopping inches from Nate's orange juice. While Jay and I waited breathlessly, Nate assumed his new big brother status, pointed his forefinger in the boy's face, and said with authority, "You go to your mother!" We exhaled with relief when the little rascal turned and did exactly as he had been told!

I hardly had time to catch my breath on another shopping trip. Jill, the children, and I were in Valley Mall approaching the clock area where people met each other or waited for friends on the heavy long green wood and iron benches. Suddenly Nate ran ahead of us and grabbed the back of a bench with both hands. When his weight tipped the heavy bench backward toward himself, we ran to avert a serious injury. Just before we arrived, a tall, dark-skinned man was there firmly holding the bench in place. Nate dropped to the floor, scared but unhurt. Then the man was gone before Jill or I could thank him. Where did he come from? Where did he go? I no longer have any doubt that small children are guarded by angels.

The first Virginia winter after several warm years in Florida had its highs and lows for the Snider family. In January, Becky awoke and looked out of her window to see her first major snowfall. "It's awesome," she breathed. Several weeks later, their rented farmhouse unexpectedly ran out of fuel for the furnace, and the delivery truck couldn't get there until the next day. So we had a pajama party at our house. After supper, Jay put a log into the fireplace; the children had baths with the little yellow duck, green frog, and Beatrix Potter washcloths, and we all enjoyed the relaxed warmth of the living room fire while we read bedtime stories. My journal says, "Little Tim smiled and waved bye-bye and enjoyed the hummingbird wind chime in the kitchen. Becky (a first grader) is now reading above the fourth grade level and recently got another good report card. Nate loves Richard Scarry books." Before daylight the next morning, Nate burst into our bedroom announcing a pillow fight!

In March of that year, I needed to fly to Indiana for a quarterly in-service meeting. Jill, Nate, and Tim drove me to the Shenandoah Valley airport. I had to wait a little while before my flight, and Jill would have been happy to drop me and take Timmy home for his nap, but Nate protested vigorously. "No," insisted my three-year-old space age grandson. "I want to see Grandma blast off!"

Becky, soon to enter second grade, kept asking to sew on my sewing machine, so I invited her to spend the day with me. Before she came, I cut about twenty strips of fabric from brightly colored cotton scraps so that she could learn to sew straight seams. She set to work with delight and quickly mastered the coordination of her hands and the knee pedal of my machine. After lunch we went to Walmart to buy Veggie Tales fleece for a pillowcase and two white tee shirts to decorate with fabric markers for herself and Nate. It was a delightful day for both of us. Later she sent this e-mail:

Dear Grandma,

I love you. When can we have another sewing lesson? How is work today?
Do you like your new car?
This is a song for you:
There are seven continents,
I can name them all:
Asia, Africa, Australia, Antarctica, North America, South America,
Europe, too.
I can name the continents.
How about you?

Love,
Becky

Christmas 2001 was coming, and the American Girl doll catalogs had arrived in every little girl's mailbox. Becky pored over her copy with longing and chose the doll she really wanted but was led to believe that these expensive dolls and their pricey accessories were out of reach. I pondered the expenditure carefully and then did the right thing. I ordered Felicity along with an extra outfit. On Christmas Day, Becky innocently opened the box and was so overcome with surprise that she sank back into the sofa pillows and let the box slide down her legs to the floor. All day, she carefully tended her new little friend from Williamsburg, and I had the happy satisfaction of money well spent.

Sometimes preschool Timmy spent several hours with me, while Jill got her hair cut or ran an errand. One afternoon, she brought him before his nap was finished. When he woke, he was startled to find himself in a different place and began to cry. At that most opportune moment, there was a loud noise outside the window. "Oh look, Timmy," I said. "Look at this street sweeper truck!" He joined me at the window and became so fascinated with the huge revolving brushes that he gave up crying and went from window to window to watch the big truck in action with all the noise and power a little boy loves.

On another day, I had hard-boiled some eggs and was peeling them. Timmy wanted to help, so I got a little stool, and he stood beside me at the sink. With a little misgiving, I gave him an egg, and he set to work. To my surprise, he did a perfect job! "Timmy," I praised him, "that's wonderful! Thank you so much!" He looked up at me and paused briefly, while the little wheels in his head brought back the appropriate rejoinder. "The pleasure was all mine!" he said.

On his fifth birthday, Timmy spent the morning with Jay and me, while Jill went with Nate on a field trip. First, we went to Milky Way Farm and rode the wagon into the strawberry patch where Timmy ate so many berries, dirt and all, that I worried about his tummy. Then he made friends with a hopping toad that entertained him until we finished our picking. After that, we went to Walmart to find a birthday present. His grandpa and I steered him toward the toys, but he wanted to see the fish. Finally, we bought a blue and purple betta with long filmy fins, a little tank, and some fish food. Timmy was so happy he made up a sweet song that he sang in the backseat all the way to Broadway. "I love you, Rainbow," he sang to his fish over and over as we drove home.

One Valentine's Day, we mailed invitations to Becky, Nate, and Tim for a pizza supper and Valentine party at our house, while Jill and Craig had an evening out. The children came, wearing red as they had been instructed, and began to hunt the little lollipops Grandpa Jay had hidden in the living room. After supper, we all began to rehearse our play, "Little Red Riding Hood," for performance later in the evening when the parents returned. The play booklet had punch-out masks for Little Red Riding Hood (Becky), the wolf (Nate), the woodcutter (Tim), and the grandmother (Peggy). Jay wore his beret, and both narrated and directed the show which was an acclaimed success!

Sometimes the creative activity was initiated by the grandchildren. While Jill and Craig went Christmas shopping one Saturday, Becky, Nate, and Tim spent the afternoon with us. They came well prepared with the handmade money and products necessary to play "store." After they set up their "shops," we were issued our money. Becky's dress shop invited us to vote for one of three dresses which she then modeled for us. She also offered nail treatments. For "five dollars," I got my nails polished purple! Nate had creepy crawlers cut from yarn which cost "one dollar" for five. Tim had a zoo of his stuffed animals for sale. He accepted our "money" but made it clear that we understood that we had to give his animals back! After we had pretty much exhausted our monetary resources, they suggested that *I* open a "café" and sell *them* ice cream sandwiches!

While the children were still small, we enjoyed several visits to Washington DC. On her first trip, Becky claimed to "extremely, extremely, extremely" love the Metro train and said she wished she could ride it to church every Sunday! On another visit, Nate's fascination with the escalators far exceeded his interest in the exhibits at the museum. We visited the zoo several times, but it was our special privilege to take the children for their first visit to the National Gallery of Art. It was a beautiful balmy day in March, and lots of people were flying kites on the mall. After we enjoyed the outdoor sculpture garden, we climbed up the long steps of the west building, passed Mercury among his huge marble columns, and found the larger-than-life painting of "Daniel in the Lion's Den" by Rubens. Downstairs, we ate lunch and enjoyed the "wall of water" before taking the moving sidewalk to the east building and the contemporary collection. Here, the bright colors, innovative techniques, and modern designs seemed to speak the language of our contemporary grandchildren. On the way back to the Metro, we rode the prancing horses of the carousel on the mall which was Timmy's favorite activity.

These stories could continue—stories of the origin of Becky's swan collection, of carving pumpkins and making applesauce, of children's choir concerts, piano recitals, drawing lessons, geography bees, costumes for *The King and I*, the annual Christmas gift "inventories," birthday dinners, flutes, LEGO kits, Redskin jerseys, Easter clothing, and holiday meals. "It is so wonderful to have your grandchildren close by," people often tell me wistfully, and I certainly do agree.

What will Becky, Nate, and Tim remember from these early years, and what will "childhood amnesia" erase? What do I hope they will remember? I have considered that question and decided, if given only one memory of these years with their grandparents, I would hope that they will remember the dining room table. This is where family life is often at its best. I hope they will retain a visual image of the table itself, set with a blue or red cloth, decorated with Jay's roses in season, napkins to mark the occasion—birthday, valentine, Thanksgiving, multicolored goblets at Christmastime—and appetizing food. I want them to remember holding hands around the table and singing our thanks together. I want them to remember where they always sat—Grandpa Jay at the head with Tim to his right and Nate to his left. Becky's chair was on my left at the end nearest the kitchen. I want them to remember a grandmother who loved to cook for her family.

I invited each grandchild to suggest a food they like to include with this entry. The survey response came back: Tim (age ten), salmon; Becky (age sixteen), "that blueberry cream cheese French toast thing"; and Nate (age thirteen), poppy seed salad dressing!

BAKED SALMON FILETS DIJON (Tim's Choice)

4 (4 ounces each) fillets salmon
2 tablespoons Dijon mustard
¼ cup dry bread crumbs or panko
¼ cup butter
Salt and pepper to taste

Preheat oven to 400 degrees. Line an eleven-by-seven-inch baking pan with foil. Place each fillet on top of foil, skin side down. Spread a thin layer of Dijon-style mustard on the top of each fillet. Cover the mustard layer with bread crumbs or panko. Drizzle butter over the tops of the fillets. Season with salt and pepper. Bake for fifteen minutes or until fillets flake easily with a fork. Makes four servings.

Or if you prefer:

Prepare salmon fillets without the Dijon and crumbs. Glaze with melted butter or olive oil before baking. Season. Serve with sour cream dill sauce.

Sour Cream Dill Sauce

⅓ cup sour cream
3 tablespoons mayonnaise or salad dressing
1 tablespoon fresh dill chopped (or ¾ teaspoon dried dill)

BLUEBERRY-STUFFED FRENCH TOAST (Becky's Choice)

1 large loaf French bread
1 (8 ounce) package cream cheese
1 cup fresh or frozen blueberries
12 eggs, beaten
2 cups milk
⅓ cup maple syrup
¼ teaspoon cinnamon

Cut bread into one-inch cubes and place half in a nine-by-thirteen-inch baking dish. Partially freeze cream cheese before cutting one-fourth-inch slices to spread over bread crumbs. Sprinkle the blueberries over the bread and cheese and add other half of crumbs. Mix eggs, milk, cinnamon, and maple syrup. Pour over bread mixture. Chill overnight. Remove from refrigerator thirty minutes before baking. Bake at 350 degree for thirty minutes covered. Then uncover and bake for another thirty minutes until firm. Slice and serve with warm maple syrup.

POPPY SEED SALAD DRESSING (Nate's Choice)

¼ cup white vinegar
⅔ cup of sugar
2 teaspoons prepared mustard
1 teaspoon grated onion
¼ teaspoon salt
¾ cup canola oil
1 teaspoon poppy seeds

In a blender, combine the vinegar, sugar, mustard, onion, and salt; cover and process until well blended. While processing, gradually add oil in a steady stream. Stir in poppy seeds.

(Option 1) *Swiss Cashew Tossed Salad*
1 medium bunch romaine lettuce, torn into bite-sized pieces
2 stalks sliced celery and/or one half red pepper slivered
1 cup cashew halves
4 ounces Swiss cheese, julienned

(Option 2) *Mandarin Strawberry Salad*
4 cups romaine lettuce, torn into bite-sized pieces
4 cups baby spinach, torn
4 cups red cabbage, thinly sliced
1 eleven-ounce can mandarin orange sections, drained
1 and ½ cups strawberries, quartered
Several slices red onion, separated into rings (optional)

GRANDPARENTS HEATWOLE

Abram Daniel (1872-1939) and Lydia Ellen (Heatwole) (1875-1949) Heatwole

Granddaddy Heatwole died of tuberculosis at age sixty-seven when I was two months old. My parents told me that he held me briefly soon after my birth and said, "A fine baby girl." With that blessing, I have tried to reconstruct a picture of my grandfather and his life from a few memories of stories from my parents and by reading between the lines of those who have written briefly about him.

Harry A. Brunk, historian, (*David Heatwole and His Descendants*, Park View Press, 1987) records that Abram was a *fifth* generation American. His ancestor Johann Mathias Hutwohl (1711-1776) left his home in Steeg, Germany, to seek religious freedom and a better life in the New World. Mathias landed at Philadelphia in 1748 after a turbulent voyage on the ship *Two Brothers* during which he lost his wife and two small daughters. After several years in the new world, he married a Ms. Haas and had six children.

David Heatwole (1767-1842), first son of Mathias and Ms. Haas and *first* generation American, married Magdalene Weyland who, as a young woman, had escaped an Indian massacre that destroyed her home by lying flat in the bottom of a canoe and floating downstream. With the promise of cheap, fertile land in Virginia, David and his family moved by wagon team in the spring of 1797. He was a farmer, a shoemaker, and the first deacon in the Virginia Mennonite Church.

Gabriel Heatwole (1789-1875), son of David and *second* generation American, married Margaret (Polly) Swank, and they were blessed with twelve children. Gabriel and Polly settled in the woods at the base of Mole Hill where they labored to clear and farm a huge tract of land. "Doc" Gabriel was a Thomasonian country doctor who advocated natural remedies. He also owned a sawmill and worked as a cooper. Brunk says many antiques treasured today by Rockingham County folks, including split bottom chairs, were made in the cooper shop by Gabriel and his employees. (Were the five split bottom chairs that were used in the Heatwole homestead for many years and which I inherited from my father made in Gabriel's shop? It is a good possibility!) In 1832, Gabriel built a new house in front of his old log cabin with walls five bricks thick that is now recognized by his progeny as the Heatwole homestead.

Gabriel and Polly's son, John G. Heatwole (1816-1869), *third* generation American, married Elizabeth Rhodes. Their son Manassas was two years old when his mother died.

Manassas Heatwole (1843-1890), *fourth* generation American, had the red hair which occasionally flames again in succeeding generations. Exciting stories are told of his activities during the Civil War from which he was listed on the Consolidated Roll of Rebel Deserters. He married Margaret Weaver, and they had nine children, of which Abram (my grandfather) was the third child and first son. This family owned the Gabriel Heatwole homestead and farmed its land in the shadow of Mole Hill.

What was life like for young Abram in those early years after the Civil War? Certainly, he heard his father, Manassas, a man of faith who was opposed to war, tell stories of his attempt to escape to the North, his capture and imprisonment, his forced induction into the Confederate Army, and his desertion. Certainly, Abram looked in wonder at the concealed trapdoor in the closet of his home which allowed his fugitive father to drop into the crawl space if any stranger on horseback approached.

After the Civil War, life began to change for many in the United States with the industrial development of the North, the taming of the West, and the rise of a new South. Many American families left their farms and moved to cities, and railroads created national markets. Retail selling, once handled by peddlers and general stores, became big business in the late 1800s.

However, Abram's early life was not affected drastically by these developments. When farm chores were done, he accompanied his father on horseback to Minnick's (later Whitmore's) General Merchandise Store and Post Office at Dale Enterprise to pick up the mail and purchase a few things on Mother Margaret's store list. Nancy Hess (*By the Grace of God,* Park View Press, 1979, p. 148) describes "this friendly store with its checker-paned windows, high front porch, and bell-tingling door; the dark interior smelled like coffee beans, raw leather, and pickled herring. Almost anything could be found here—from saddles to soap, to hats and shoes and thread, to cough syrup for people, to liniment for horses, to great wheels of longhorn cheese." Here too, young Abram listened to the men of the community who gathered around the woodstove to sort out the political troubles of Presidents Ulysses S. Grant, Rutherford B. Hayes, and James A. Garfield.

The public school system expanded swiftly in the late 1800s as the United States sought to become the first nation to educate its entire population. Young Abram attended Paul's Summit School located on Silver Lake Road near Dayton, Virginia. Many small one- or two-room schools dotted Rockingham County at that time, making it possible for children to walk to a school where they could receive the basic tools to become literate adults.

New inventions began to bring a new way of life to Americans, although they were sometimes slow in coming to country people. When Abram was three years old (1875), the first telephone was invented. Later in his life, when the first telephone lines were strung through the Mole Hill section, Abram used his team of horses to haul chestnut trees out of the Shenandoah Mountains to be used for poles. When Abram was seven years old (1879),

Thomas Edison succeeded in placing a filament of carbonized thread in a bulb that burned all night. It would be several years yet before electricity lighted Abram's home, and oil lamps were no longer needed.

The Heatwole family faithfully attended Weavers Mennonite Church. H. D. Weaver (*Christian Monitor*, September 1932) wrote an article about the history of this church. He says, "The first revival was held at Weavers in December 1888 by John S. Coffman who came from the West and preached one whole week at night. Although there was much objection to this apparent innovation, yet the spirit of the Lord worked mightily during the series of meetings that resulted in forty-four converts who were baptized on December 30, and from which number came many of the prominent workers of the Church today." Abram D. Heatwole's name appears on the list. He was fifteen years old at this time and remained a member at Weavers throughout his life.

Romance blossomed when Abram became of age, and the object of his affection was Lydia Ellen Heatwole who lived with her family on a nearby farm. Lydia was the daughter of Peter S. Heatwole who was a first cousin to Manassas.

As a young man, Lydia's father, Peter Heatwole, reluctantly enlisted in the Confederate Army as a teamster. After a year, he became so disgusted with the awfulness of war that he handed the reins of the horses he had led for a drink at the bank of the Potomac River near Williamsport, Maryland, to another man, jumped into the water, and swam across the Potomac to freedom.

Under cover of night, he walked six miles until he met a Mennonite farmer, John Reiff, near Hagerstown who gave him food, introduced Peter to his wife and pretty fourteen-year-old daughter Nancy, and gave him work on his farm. A little over a year later, Peter and Nancy were married and set up housekeeping on one side of the double-occupancy brick Reiff home. The young couple was happy on the Reiff farm, but when the war was over, Peter, homesick for his valley home, convinced Nancy to move to Virginia with him. Lydia Ellen was the fifth child in Peter and Nancy's family of seven.

Abram and Lydia were married April 12, 1894. Their formal wedding picture portrays a twenty-two-year-old man comfortably seated in his wicker armchair, left leg over right knee, wearing a dark suit with satin edging on the collar, winged shirt collar, and wide tie. His nineteen-year-old dark-haired bride stands gracefully by his side, hand on the back of the wicker chair. She is fashionably attired in a long dark dress with white bow, puffed sleeves, tightly corseted waist, and skirt with a bustle. Lydia's father and mother gave her a cookstove and a dough tray as a wedding gift. They lived on the one-hundred-one-acre Heatwole homestead which they purchased from the

Manassas Heatwole Estate in 1904 for four thousand five hundred dollars. My father, Roy Abram, was second to last of their ten children.

In addition to the heavy demands of farm work, Abram was often involved in community activities. He was a member of the Dale Enterprise School Board, served as a poll judge on election days, and was a member of the executive committee of the Shenandoah Stockmen's Association. Abram was always interested and active in politics. I was startled in my college American History class when Professor Harry Brunk announced to me and all my classmates that my grandfather Heatwole *always* voted the Democratic ticket.

Each May, Abram, on his favorite horse, Fancy, and other men and boys of the Dale Enterprise community, rounded up their cattle and drove them cowboy-style to a cattle camp in the mountains west of Dayton at Hone Quarry, a two- or three-day's journey on horseback. There, Abram's herd, branded with a "D" on the left hip, grazed for a small price until October. The Heatwole family and their friends enjoyed many good times hiking, wading in the creek, pitching horseshoes, and simply relaxing at the cattle camp.

Heartbreak struck the Heatwole home in January 1919 when two members of the family died in the epidemic of Spanish influenza. In December, when the disease seemed to have loosened its grip on the Valley, the Heatwole family decided to attend a Christmas program at the Dale Enterprise School. Soon after, the flu flared again, and daughters, Annie, age twenty-one, and Mary, age eighteen and soon to be married, died on two consecutive days. My father, Roy, a three-year-old, appeared to be sicker than his sisters but recovered. A nurse who was caring for the family, Mollie Wenger, also became ill and died at the Heatwole home.

In 1920, Abram and his brother John G. visited a friend in Steamboat Springs, Colorado, where they rode a steam engine to Pike's Peak. Abram remarked that he would rather drive a steam engine than be president of the United States! His wish was granted when he and five of his friends formed a steam engine company and did custom work in the Dale Enterprise community. His children remember that one of his favorite early morning activities was firing up the steam engine to build its head of steam for the day's work.

Henry Ford pioneered in the assembly line production of automobiles, and by 1916, the Model T could be bought for less than four hundred dollars. Sometime later, Abram owned a Dodge automobile which he nicknamed "D. B." after the Dodge Brothers who manufactured it. My father recalled that Granddaddy Abram had some trouble driving "D. B." and making the shift from the steam engine and his two-horse surrey!

Abram was a good-humored man who loved a joke and didn't mind when the joke was on him. Once when he drove his car down to Dayton on an errand, he thought he saw his beloved border collie, Jack, on the street, so he picked up the dog and put him in the car. When he arrived home, he was surprised to see his Jack come running up to greet him! He quickly got into his car and hurried to drive the other dog back to Dayton!

Music made Heatwole family life and its routines more enjoyable. Abram and his daughters often sang together as they milked the cows. He played "Soldier's Joy" on the French harp, and one of his favorite songs was "Red Wing," the sad story of a pretty Indian maid who lost her lover brave.

> Now the moon shines tonight on pretty Red Wing—
> The breeze is sighing; the night bird's crying—
> For afar 'neath his star her brave is sleeping—
> While Red Wing's weeping her heart away.

Grandma Lydia's 1860 edition of the *Harmonia Sacra* indicates that she owned a book and enjoyed attending hymn sings, probably including the annual New Year's Day Hymn Sing at Weavers which began in 1903. A penciled autograph jingle and the name of A. D. Heatwole on the inside cover suggests that her mind wandered occasionally to her lover!

> "YY you are; YY you be—(Two y's/Too wise . . .)
> I see you are YY for me!"

Abram and Lydia and five of their children are pictured on the 1924 long photograph of the Dale Enterprise Literary Society Reunion. This society met every Friday evening to enjoy recitations and pantomimes and to hold spelling bees and singings.

Hard times struck the Heatwole family again in 1927 when the excellent herd of dairy cattle that produced a good income for the family contracted "Bang's Disease" or tuberculosis, and many had to be destroyed. Two years later in 1929, the stock market crashed, and the country sank into a deep depression. Banks failed. Farm prices fell lower than ever before. In September 1930, a son-in-law returned from Dayton with the news that the bank had closed. Finding that news hard to believe, Abram drove to Dayton only to find out for himself that the report was true. The closing came at a hard time for all the area farmers who needed to buy their winter's supply of feed and seeds. When the bank's accounts were finalized, each person with an account there received eleven cents on the dollar.

Even though times were hard, there was one thing the Heatwole family never lacked—good food—and plenty of it. Grandma Lydia was a warm and gentle mother who successfully managed her household in a way that was both economical and abundant. Lydia's mother, Nancy Reiff, from Maryland "brought more to Virginia than her mother's possessions. She brought a whole new way of life: interesting customs, colorful Deutsch speech, a variety of talents and new ideas, different methods of gardening, preparing food, and tasty German dishes with lots of vinegar and spices, sassy sayings, and old German proverbs" (Hess, p. 139).

Lydia learned her mother's ways of housekeeping, including the tradition of seven sweets and seven sours to round out her abundant meals. Her daughter-in-law, my mother, often recalled Lydia's extensive company menus which might include mashed potatoes, sweet potatoes, potato salad, and some twenty or more other items in the same meal. Once the dining table, too heavily laden with food, literally broke just before the crew of silo fillers came in from the fields for dinner, spilling food onto the floor and delaying the meal while new preparations were made.

My mother made a deliciously rich soup called "Spotsie Pot Pie" that she learned from Grandma Lydia. It had sausage, potatoes, and rivels (dry crumbles made with egg and flour) but was made without a written recipe, so it now lives only in my memory as one of my favorite soups.

After Abram's death in 1939, my Uncle George and family moved into the homestead with Grandma Lydia. She lived on for ten years before her death in 1949 from diabetes and its complications. My family visited her often on Sunday afternoons. Even so, my memories of her, sitting quietly in her chair, are quite dim, probably because I spent most of my time playing outside with my cousin Paul on the long sidewalk that led to the milk house where we dabbled in the troughs filled with cold water from the well. I was Lydia's eighteenth grandchild, so perhaps the thrill of having new grandchildren had blunted over the years, or maybe she was just tired from preparing all those huge meals over a lifetime.

I do have one very tangible point of connection with Grandma Lydia Ellen. Before my birth, she told my parents if they had a girl, and if they named her Ellen, she would give that granddaughter the set of six cups and saucers she herself had inherited as a namesake. My belief is that this set had been given to her by her aunt, Lydia Ann (Heatwole) Grove, a sister of Peter S. Heatwole, her father. Lydia Ann birthed no children of her own, and so she gave them to her niece and namesake.

The saucer-bowls of the set are deep for cooling a hot beverage; the small cups are without handles. They are translucent china and decorated with a pale blue-green border of stars and vines. When did Lydia Ann, born in the early 1800s, receive these lovely dishes? Who were the prior owners? How fortunate I have been to be entrusted by my grandmother, whose name I carry, to be their caretaker on their journey through time.

(I am grateful for the informational items in the collection of family stories gathered by Sandra Heatwole and edited by Scott Suter, *History of Abram D. Heatwole of Rocky Hollow*, Park View Press, 1988.)

In the Heatwole family, there is one food essential to every important occasion or family reunion, and that is sugar-cured country ham. Here are several ways to bring this revered regional specialty to the table.

SUGAR-CURED COUNTRY HAM

To prepare ham

Scrub ham well with warm water to remove curing material and mold bloom. *Do this for all four methods listed below.* (Mold is normal for country-cured hams.)

Soaking to remove some of the salt is optional to taste. The ham may be soaked three or four hours or overnight, as desired. Discard soaking water.

To pan fry ham slices

Slice ham one-fourth inch thick. Trim rind.

Roll slices of ham in flour, shaking off excess.

Grease skillet lightly. Start with a cold skillet and fry on low heat, turning ham frequently, until slices are delicately browned.

To boil ham

Trim off rind and excessive fat, or if you prefer, the rind may be removed after cooking.

Cover ham with water, add one-fourth cup vinegar, and heat to boiling. Reduce heat, and simmer twenty minutes per pound, or use meat thermometer to 160 degrees. Remove kettle from heat, and allow ham to cool in broth. Remove ham from broth, and cool in the refrigerator for easier slicing.

To bake ham

Place ham on rack in roasting pan, fat side up. Pour two cups of water in bottom of roaster. Cover roaster and bake for twenty minutes per pound at 325 degrees, or use meat thermometer to 160 degrees.

Ham may be served hot or cold.

To bake ham slices

Cut ham slices one-half inch thick. Sprinkle with brown sugar and dry mustard.

Place slices flat in a large baking dish. Cover ham with milk and bake at 325 degrees for forty-five minutes.

Do not discard the bone! Our ancestors would have used it to make a delicious bean soup!

GRANDPARENTS SUTER

Lawrence Emanuel (1891-1964) and Emma Pearl (Showalter) (1890-1947) Suter

It was 1960, and I was a junior in college when I learned about the eleven-week European Student Tour arranged by Menno Travel Service. The cost was a little over one thousand dollars, a staggering amount for a student then but would hardly buy the airfare today. A note from the MTS director reminded would-be travelers that "it has not been so long when few people had the opportunity to visit another country. Most of your parents have only dreamed of going abroad." How much less our grandparents!

With some hesitancy, but no real fear, I went to visit my grandfather, Lawrence Emanuel Suter, in his office at the Harrisonburg warehouse where he sold feed and fertilizer to farmers. He was seated at his dusty desk. He was a portly man with thinning grey hair and friendly blue eyes wearing a khaki work shirt buttoned to the neck with a pen and little black notebook in the left pocket. "Granddaddy," I began, "I need to borrow a thousand dollars." He may have looked a bit startled by my announcement, but he waited for me to explain, and when he had heard my story, he granted my request without reserve and with no interest added. His generosity, a signature characteristic of L. E. Suter, and his trust in me established a lifetime of gratitude from his granddaughter.

Later that summer in Switzerland, our tour took us to a place where early Anabaptists worshiped and were buried, and I saw the name "Sutter" on a gravestone.

The original home of the Suter family was in the beautiful village of Kolliken in the Canton Aargau of Switzerland. In 1539, the government of Bern ordered a survey of all arable land at Kolliken. Six Suters were among the tenants and had in their possession the saw mill and tannery. They were craftsmen, shoemakers (supposedly the origin of the name "Suter"), tanners, millers, and farmers. Granddaddy's ancestor, whose first name we do not know, later moved to the Alsace, Lorraine, area of France where he was a "king's weaver," possibly serving royalty there.

This man's son, John Suter, married Barbara Christener, and they had five children, one of whom was Daniel, born October 8, 1808.

In 1826, Daniel Suter and two of his siblings immigrated to America. Daniel came to the Shenandoah Valley where he is reported to have been a man with many abilities—speaker of five languages of which his preferred was German: cabinet maker and carpenter; weaver of cloth, carpets, and fancy coverlets; and musician. He loved to walk, often arriving at church before those who drove and walked twice to Ohio to visit his brother.

Daniel married Anna Heatwole in August 1828 and settled near Dayton, Virginia. They had five children, one of whom was Emanuel, the son with whom he was living when he died in 1873 (extracted from *Memories of Yesteryear*, Mary Eugenia Suter, Charles F. McClung, Printer, 1959, pp. 1-5).

Emanuel Suter, fourth child of Daniel and Anna and *first* generation born in America, was born in 1833. His mother died of typhoid fever two years later, and he grew up in the home of his uncle, Shem Heatwole. At age eighteen, he became an apprentice to his cousin, John D. Heatwole, a potter. In 1855, Emanuel married Elizabeth Swope, and they had a family of thirteen children.

Between 1856 and 1860, Emanuel built a pottery on the farm three miles west of Harrisonburg that he and Elizabeth inherited from her father. During the Civil War, he was exempted from military service because his skills as a potter were needed to make tableware. Following the terrible raid in the Shenandoah Valley by General Sheridan, Emanuel and Elizabeth and their children fled north to Harrisburg, Pennsylvania. As he fled, Emanuel began writing a diary of his experiences which he kept on a daily basis until his death in 1902.

In addition to his pottery business, Emanuel was very active in his church and community. He served for many years on the local school board, attended court day in Harrisonburg, wrote wills, and settled estates for his neighbors. He was "a strong advocate of Sunday schools, and he did all in his power, it seems, to organize and attend Sunday schools in and outside the Mennonite Church." (*History of Mennonites in Virginia 1727-1900*, Harry A. Brunk, McClure Printing Company, 1959, p. 203)

John R. Suter, fifth child of Emanuel and Elizabeth and *second* generation born in America, was born in 1863 during the Civil War. As an infant in 1864, he was among those carried north to Pennsylvania by wagon to escape the union raids and the imposition of the confederacy. This early trauma did not seem to adversely mark his personality, and he was always known as a jolly man, easy in his relationships with other people.

In 1884, John R. married Fannie Roudabush, and they had eleven children. They lived in a dwelling on the east corner of the Suter Homestead where a post office, Suters, had opened, and Fannie served as postmistress. John R. farmed the farm and taught school at New Erection School. His niece, Mary E. Suter, tells that he had to correct his pupils so often for using "forgit" instead of "forget." One day, he very emphatically told them (and he spelled out the word) f-o-r-g-e-t spells forget and don't "forgit" it! Laughter followed, and he joined in heartily. (Suter, p. 124)

John R. owned the first Model T Ford in the Suter family. Returning home from his first driving lesson, he pulled up in front of the house to park and pushed the foot pedal down to the floor, suddenly throwing the car into low gear. The car leaped forward, took off the mailbox, and came to rest against the fence. He never drove again. Later when he became a traveling salesman, he used the train; and when he needed to make car trips, he persuaded his younger sons and grandsons to drive him where he wanted to go. He traveled throughout Virginia and West Virginia for the Johnson Harvesting Company and later for Griffith and Boyd Fertilizer Company until his death in 1945. As he grew older, he operated primarily from a warehouse in Harrisonburg.

I have a dim image of my great-grandfather sitting at his desk in the office of the warehouse. He always dressed up for work and was wearing a suit and vest with a little bowtie. As a preschool child, I approached him and told him candidly that his tie looked like Dagwood's! My mother was aghast, but I remember his chuckle.

Lawrence Emanuel Suter, fourth child of John R. and Fannie and *third* generation born in America, was born in 1891 and grew up with his seven brothers and two sisters and many other members of the Suter clan on the properties of the Suter Homestead west of Harrisonburg. He attended the two-room country school of New Erection, receiving a seventh grade education, typical at that time. In 1912, he married (Emma) Pearl Showalter, and they had four children of which the third was my mother Dorothy.

Pearl was the fourth of nine children in the family of Mary E. (Heatwole), 1862-1950, and Jacob D. Showalter (1854-1939). Pearl's paternal grandparents were John D. and Elizabeth Driver Showalter, and her maternal grandparents were Joseph and Lydia (Rhodes) Heatwole. Family lines often cross in a small sectarian community such as Rockingham County, and my great-grandmother Mary was the youngest half sister of my Heatwole grandmother Lydia! (Figure that out when you have the time!)

I fidgeted and found little to amuse myself when Mother took me to visit my great-grandmother Showalter who sat in her chair at Aunt Maud's house, nearly blind and wearing a green celluloid visor. Mother assured me that she had been the "perfect grandmother," making better chicken and homemade noodles than any other person. She had been a strong lady, the bulwark of her family. My tangible reminder of this once stately lady sits in my cupboard, an elegant cut-glass compote with fluted edge, a piece my mother treasured greatly.

Little is known about my great-granddad Showalter, a rather short and quiet man, his wife's senior by eight years. He owned a beautiful farm until a son-in-law's business venture went awry, and the note Granddad had signed had to be paid. If Grandma was known as outgoing and generous, Granddad was perhaps less so. My Uncle Richard, his young grandson, remembers riding with him to the store in Dayton. Richard stood expectantly by the ice cream chest, hoping his granddad would buy him a cone, but Granddad did not take the hint! (An aside to all grandparents—Be remembered for your generosity as I remember my Grandfather Lawrence for his loan for my European tour. Buy the American Girl Doll or the Medieval Village LEGO set; it's a small price to pay for a child's happy memory!)

The Showalter family, with six living daughters and one son, was somewhat unusual for families of their community with respect to education, especially for females. Two daughters, Margaret and Maud, with interests in art and music respectively, went to Goshen College in Indiana. My grandmother, Pearl, studied at Bridgewater College before earning her teacher's certificate at the Normal School in Harrisonburg, now James Madison University. Scarcely five feet tall, petite Pearl drove her own horse and buggy from Dayton to Harrisonburg every day to complete her education. In 1911, she began her short teaching career at Rushville School located near the Bank Mennonite Church. (Harold D. Lehman, Professor of Education Emeritus at James Madison University, recently told me that there were some two hundred one and two-room schools such as Rushville dotted over Rockingham County in the years before and after the turn of the century as the need arose to provide classrooms within walking distances. Sadly, some of these schools carried the name "Colored" since desegregation did not happen for another fifty years.)

Home life was generally happy for the Lawrence and Pearl Suter family. Granddaddy continued the feed and fertilizer business begun by his father. The hours were long, and the work was hard, but he was strong. Farmers drove their horses and wagons to Harrisonburg and waited in line for their turn to pull up to the boxcar door and be loaded. Sometimes Granddaddy carried the two-hundred-pound bags back along the line to load wagons that were in a hurry. He worked six days a week, and often on Saturdays, he would bring home a bag of candy for his four children. Sometimes they begged him to bring "store bread" instead of candy!

Recently, it was my good fortune to have a long conversation with my Uncle Richard, the only living member of that generation. Although the family lived during the days of the Depression, he said the children never felt poor; they always had enough and had plenty of food. There was a big garden, cows to milk, and hogs and chickens to butcher. Sometimes Granddaddy took a grocery list to the store in Dayton where a clerk would run around and gather up items, measure things from big glass jars, and finally tie up the package on the counter. The family celebrated Christmas with gifts, candy, and popcorn balls. Richard remembers using oil lamps and a refrigerator with blocks of ice before they had electricity. They had a "party-line" telephone that hung on the wall which rang "two longs and two shorts" for them, but it was the custom of the community to eavesdrop on all the neighbors' calls as well. Church attendance was not negotiable, alternating each Sunday between Bank Mennonite and Pike Mennonite Churches where Granddaddy often served as Sunday school superintendent. After church, company frequently came for dinner and enjoyed Grandma's tender, juicy fried chicken and dried apple pie. Richard says Grandma "rated way up there" as a good cook!

As the children began to marry, Grandma and Granddaddy helped them establish their own homes. Grandma helped Uncle Harold to place an order from the Sears and Roebuck catalog for a bed and dresser, iron range, kitchen cabinet, breakfast set, and day bed—all for the amazing price of one hundred dollars!

I was the first granddaughter following four grandsons, and that always made me feel like a special little person. When I was three and my baby brother was born, I stayed with my grandparents for a week. To amuse me, Grandma sewed clothes for my doll and told me stories. I somehow remember one little green doll dress with white polka dots that she made from an old shirt. Grandma loved to sew and quilt. I am fortunate to have a "bubble gum pink and poison green" dahlia pattern quilt she and my mother made together using popular colors of the 1930s.

When I was in the second grade, I wrote my grandma a letter and sent it by mail. I still have her sweet reply.

Dayton, Va.
January 21, 1947

Dear Peggy,

I got a letter from you today so I will write you one. I am sitting here in my rocking chair and can't write very good, but I hope you can read it. I guess you are in school reading your lesson on something. Are you good and warm when the wind is blowing so hard and cold? It was too bad I wasn't at home when you came Sunday. I hope I will be here the next time you come. Aunt Zettie and Lonnie were here a little while yesterday afternoon. Winston and Charlie were in school. I guess your doll didn't like it in school if she cried. What do you call her? Does Jimmie like to play with his scooter?

Granddaddy and Richard are in town. We will come to see you when we can.

Goodbye, from
Grandma

Later that same year, September 1947, my Grandma Suter died of breast cancer that had spread to her lungs. I remember the sadness of those days. Granddaddy chose to bring her body home, often the custom at that time.

The huge casket, with its imposing lid, stood in the parlor where friends and extended family came to pay their respects. On the morning of the funeral, we gathered for a short service at the home before the procession moved to Weavers Church for the final memorial and interment in the Weavers Cemetery.

Granddaddy's sister, Nettie, came to keep house for him and Uncle Richard after Grandma's death. Granddaddy remained a widower for seventeen years before his death in 1964. During that time, he kept busy with his business and church work, but an aura of grief sometimes surrounded him. Shortly before his death from Hodgkin's disease, Ann and Jill were born, and he held them proudly for a photograph.

Always a generous giver, Granddaddy shared his humongous tomatoes and succulent cantaloupes with neighbors and friends. One of his many Bibles, passed from Mother to me, contained numerous personal thank you notes from church leaders for his generous Christmas gifts and support of special causes.

In July 2006, Jay and I attended the John R. Suter family reunion at Laurel Lake near the foot of Shenandoah Mountain. As usual, the food was abundant, exceptionally rich, and tasty. There was plenty of fried chicken, always the Suter family favorite. Nolan Suter, a nephew of my Granddaddy Lawrence, told me a story I want to remember.

Nolan and his family had recently taken a car trip out West and stayed overnight in a motel in California. In the morning as they packed their car, a man noticed their Virginia license plate and engaged Nolan in conversation. The man had once lived in Virginia, and as part of his employment, he helped indigent families manage their debts. He asked whether Nolan might know a man named Lawrence Suter. When Nolan responded that Lawrence was his uncle, the man proceeded to tell Nolan that he had once gone to see Lawrence in his office at the warehouse about a family that was in serious financial straits. The family owed Lawrence something like four thousand dollars. Lawrence slowly leafed through a stack of accounts about an inch thick, looking at each, until he found the bill in question. Then he picked up his pen and wrote across the top "Paid in Full."

Ironically, the sermon I had heard in church that very morning was about greed, one of the "Seven Deadly Sins." How wonderful, I reflected, to be known forty years after death for generosity rather than for having four thousand more dollars in your estate!

"Chicken doesn't taste as good as it used to," my uncle complained. "That's true," I replied, "and the chicken doesn't think his food tastes as good as it used to either!" For better tasting and more healthful meat, the way the Suters enjoyed it so much at home and at reunions, it may be worth paying a bit more for a free range or organic chicken which has been raised without antibiotics, pesticides, and herbicides.

SKILLET-FRIED CHICKEN

3 to 3 and ½ lbs. broiler-fryer chicken, cut into serving pieces
½ cup all-purpose flour
1 teaspoon paprika
½ teaspoon salt
¼ teaspoon pepper
Vegetable oil to cover bottom of skillet

In a plastic bag, combine flour, paprika, salt, and pepper. Rinse chicken and pat until almost dry. Shake a piece or two at a time in the plastic bag to coat.

Heat oil in a twelve-inch skillet over medium heat. Place chicken pieces in the skillet, meaty pieces toward the center, being careful not to crowd them in the pan.

Cook, uncovered, for fifteen minutes, turning pieces to brown evenly.

For a *crisp* fried chicken, continue to cook in the skillet, uncovered, over medium low heat for thirty-five to forty-five minutes or until no longer pink. Drain on paper towels.

For a *tender* fried chicken, remove pieces and arrange them skin side up in a baking pan. Place in a 375-degree oven and bake uncovered for thirty-five to forty-five minutes or until no longer pink. Do not turn.

Serves six.

The skin on the chicken and the frying oil produce a dish that is high in fat content. By removing the skin and oven-frying, one can serve a healthier version of this classic dish.

Panko (Japanese breadcrumbs) produces a very crispy oven-fried chicken and is worth a trip to an Asian market, if necessary.

OVEN-FRIED CHICKEN

⅓ cup low-fat buttermilk
2 teaspoons salt-free Cajun seasoning (optional)
½ teaspoon salt
1 cup panko (Japanese breadcrumbs)
6 meaty pieces of broiler-fryer chicken (breasts, legs, thighs), skin removed
Cooking spray

Combine buttermilk, seasoning, and salt in a shallow dish.

Place panko in a separate shallow dish.

Dip chicken one piece at a time in buttermilk. Dredge in panko.

Place chicken pieces on a baking sheet coated with cooking spray.

Lightly coat chicken with cooking spray to produce a nicely browned crust.

Bake at 400 degrees for forty to forty-five minutes, turning once after twenty minutes.

Serves four to six.

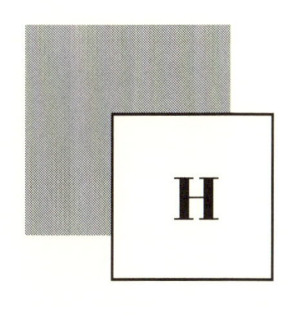

H \'āch\ (also h)
n. (pl. hs or h's)
the eighth letter of the alphabet

HOME

Recipe: Turkey and Squash Soup

Recipe: Turkey Curry

HOME

Rockingham County, in the central Shenandoah Valley of Virginia, has been my home for almost all of my life. The northern cardinal, the Virginia State Bird that is also a permanent resident of Rockingham County, loves his habitat and marks his territory with song. During courtship, the perky red male feeds seed to the female beak-to-beak. Then the female chooses a dense shrub and builds a cup nest from thin twigs and bark strips and lines it with grasses. Like the cardinals, I love my habitat—its people, history, and natural beauty. Nesting is important too. Together, they shape my concept of "home."

Virginia Governor Alexander Spotswood and his party of forty or fifty men on horseback were some of the first white people to see the land that would be called Rockingham County. Traveling from Williamsburg in the summer of 1716, they arrived at the crest of the Blue Ridge Mountains and looked down into the lush Shenandoah Valley below.

In celebration of their discovery, they jubilantly drank to the health of King George I and nicknamed themselves the "Knights of the Golden Horseshoe." After returning to Williamsburg, Governor Spotswood wrote the King, requesting a grant for the "Order of the Knights of the Golden Horseshoe." King George graciously complied and sent back the proclamation along with fifty tiny golden horseshoes. Governor Spotswood then presented each member of his expedition with a golden horseshoe inscribed:

Sic jurat transcendere montes.
(Thus he declares to climb the mountains.)

Rockingham County was established in 1777 and named in honor of a British prime minister, Charles Watson-Wintworth, the Marquees of Rockingham, a keen supporter of constitutional rights for the colonists.

My earliest Heatwole ancestor moved to Rockingham County from Pennsylvania twenty years later in 1797. By 1816, his son Gabriel had purchased a large tract of land, approximately three thousand acres, and settled in a simple log dwelling at the foot of Mole Hill. As Gabriel Heatwole's family and his finances increased, he desired a more substantial dwelling; and in 1832, he built a new house with walls five bricks thick made from the dead grass and red earth found and fired in his east meadow. The house had two large chimneys, high ceilings, and four beautiful pine-paneled fireplaces.

A few years later, he enlarged the original house with four more rooms of brick, two chimneys, and a frame summer kitchen with herb drying room. This house stands strong, awaiting its two hundredth birthday and is known as the

"Heatwole Homestead" to Gabriel's many progeny. It is the farmhouse where my father, Roy Abram Heatwole, was born in 1915 and grew to adulthood.

Pleasant Valley, My First Home

Pleasant Valley is one of the numerous small, unincorporated settlements that dot the map of Rockingham County. In 1874, the railroad came to this area, and the depot, named Pleasant Valley in recognition of this beautiful fertile area, was part of the rail line connecting Harrisonburg and Staunton.

My mother and father bought a twenty-seven-acre farm near Pleasant Valley after their marriage in 1938 and began housekeeping. I was born in the small farmhouse in 1939 and lived there until I was about three years old. I have no memories of those early years, only my mother's stories of a house with no modern conveniences but with peaceful surroundings and friendly neighbors.

Several years ago, Jay and I went searching for this house. When we believed we had located the place, we found by happenstance that an auction was in progress. Personal items were laid out on wagon beds, and pieces of furniture sat on the lawn waiting their turn on the block. We realized that the house itself was empty and open, so we stealthily entered. It was small, two-storied, with several rooms up and down and an antiquated kitchen. "Which room was I born in?" I asked the empty walls covered with yellowing wallpaper, but they kept their secret. Nothing visible suggested my advent into the community of Pleasant Valley.

Keezletown, My Childhood Home

Another small town from my past, the picturesque hamlet of Keezletown, lies at the base of Massanutten Peak. Nearby, Massanutten Caverns were discovered in 1892 when workers blasting for limestone discovered the fairyland of strange rooms and formations. In time, accommodations at the caverns included a golf course, swimming pool, lodge, and overnight cabins. A nearby trail leading up to Massanutten Peak has long attracted hikers to the area.

My father and mother bought a forty-four-acre farm three miles north of Keezletown on Indian Trail Road in the early 1940s. Our one-storied white bungalow had porches on three sides—a front porch we seldom used that stretched veranda style across the width of the house, a smaller side porch where company usually entered, and a big screened porch outside the kitchen door that provided an extension to our summer living space. This house had more conveniences, including hot and cold running water, an indoor bathroom, and a hot air furnace.

The appliances were not modern by today's standards; Mother used a wringer-type washing machine and hung everything on the clothesline to dry. The cookstove was a wood-burning range with a "warming closet" where we kept the crackers and with a hot water tank on one side. We used an iron handle to lift the round burners in order to add more firewood. The stove kept the kitchen warm and cozy, and its oven turned out wonderful cookies for after-school snacks. My own bedroom had a sunny south window and space to play with my dolls.

Mount Clinton, My Farm Home

The little village of Mount Clinton sits along the banks of never-failing Muddy Creek surrounded by sloping hills. In the 1890s, the village came into local prominence as the location of West Central Academy, a boarding school with a girls' and a boys' dormitory and a classroom building that offered a high school education. After 1902, the academy was taken into the Rockingham County School System and became Mount Clinton High School. In 1952, I spent half of my seventh grade in a newer building of Mount Clinton High School. The following school year (1952-1953), the high school grades were transferred to the new consolidated Turner Ashby High School in Dayton, Virginia.

The eighty-acre farm my father and mother bought in 1951 was located west of Harrisonburg and north of Mount Clinton on Skye Road. The farm operation included the sale of A-grade milk and eggs from commercial-laying hens. The two-storied farmhouse had five large bedrooms, kitchen, living room, dining room, bath, and laundry room. We sanded the floors, painted or papered the walls, and bought additional furniture before we moved. My bedroom upstairs had new blue wallpaper with yellow flowers and yellow curtains at the windows, the colors of my choosing. Mother loved her blue-and-white kitchen with an electric stove and other conveniences.

Park View, Our Three Homes

Jay and I have lived in Park View, a suburb of Harrisonburg, most of the years since our marriage in 1961. Jay's long tenure on the faculty of Eastern Mennonite High School, College, and University has made Park View a most convenient location. During this time, we have lived at three addresses, all within three blocks of each other!

We came home from our honeymoon to our freshly painted apartment on Park Road in the basement of the John and Emma Horst house. For a monthly rent of approximately forty dollars, we had a cozy place to relax from our teaching jobs. The fee covered most utilities and the wisdom of the landlady who instructed the new bride in matters such as the best way to pin clothes on the line to dry!

When Ann and Jill were born about two and a half years later, the apartment became a little too cozy! Our small bedroom was wall-to-wall furniture with two cribs and baby dresser, our bed and dressers, and a rocking chair.

One evening in late 1963, Monroe and Dora Wyse, who lived on Parkway Drive in the block above ours, came to visit and said they were selling their house and moving to Pennsylvania. They wondered if we might be interested in buying a home of our own. Were we interested! We went to see the little white three-bedroom bungalow, each carrying a baby in our arms.

They were asking $15,500 for what looked like an answer to prayer and what now sounds like a steal! We were struggling financially with Jay's modest salary and my part-time Latin teaching, a sitter to pay, and baby formula to buy. But with a loan from Eastern Mennonite College and Jay's father's cosignature on a bank loan, we moved ahead. We sold the lot we had bought earlier and used that money for rugs, dining room furniture, and a breakfast set.

I think of our first home with some nostalgia. As we greeted each morning, the sun came up over Massanutten Peak and streamed through our dining room window. We decorated the living-dining room in Early American style, which was popular at the time, with two large braided rugs. As a young homemaker, I was flattered when Home Economics Professor Mary Emma Showalter asked to bring her class to see our house as an example of how young people can decorate simply but attractively.

We owned this house twenty-five years until Ann and Jill had graduated from college. During that time, we lived out-of-state twice. We made improvements in the kitchen, converted the garage below into a family room, and built a wrap-around deck and patio. In 1989, we sold the property for ninety-seven thousand dollars.

One block further up the hill on Hillcrest Drive, Ira and Mary Emma Eby were selling their house and moving to a retirement community. Would we like to see their home before they put it into the hands of a realtor? "I'll go," I told Jay, "but I know I'm not interested." We owned a lot on College Avenue and had already talked to an architect about a plan we liked.

The longer we deliberated, the more it seemed like the right thing to do. The house was already built and built very well. Its living space was large enough to invite student groups, and there were two apartments below for supplemental income. "Location, location, location," the realtors say so often, and indeed, that was the chief asset—the view to the East took in the city of Harrisonburg backed by the Massanutten Range and the pale blue, Blue Ridge off in the distance. Who could say no to that!

We redecorated the interior and moved on our anniversary, June 10, 1989. That day, our new magnolia tree opened several of its creamy white blossoms.

Drivers crossing the Rockingham County line either from U.S. 11 South or the County line from U.S. 11 North are greeted by a statue of a bronze tom turkey with tail feathers fanned out, standing on top of a pyramidal limestone base with a plaque that reads "Welcome to Rockingham County—Turkey Capital." On the opposite side of the base is a plaque inscribed with the date 1955 and the names of poultry businesses and growers who donated money for the monuments.

The idea came from ten-year-old Gerald Harris who won first place in a contest sponsored by the Spotswood Garden Club in 1951. The sculptor, Carl Roseberg, a professor at William and Mary, spent five hundred hours modeling the turkey in plaster, and the Bronze Works Company of New York cast them in bronze. The turkeys are three feet tall, and their limestone bases are five feet tall. Rockingham County is the leader in Virginia in poultry production.

I have chosen to include *two* excellent recipes using turkey, one in honor of each of these magnificent sculptures!

TURKEY AND SQUASH SOUP

2 teaspoons canola oil
Small onion, chopped
1 red bell pepper, chopped
3 cloves garlic, minced
4 cups reduced-sodium chicken broth
1 small butternut squash, peeled, seeded, and cut into one-inch cubes
1 and ½ teaspoons ground cumin
2 cups diced, cooked turkey (or raw turkey cutlets cut into narrow strips)
2 cups frozen corn kernels
2 tablespoons lime juice
½ teaspoon crushed red pepper
Salt and pepper to taste

1. Heat oil in a Dutch oven or large soup kettle over medium-high heat. Add onion and bell pepper; cook, stirring often, until the vegetables begin to soften. Add garlic and cook, stirring, for one minute more. Stir in broth, squash, and cumin; cover and bring to a boil. Reduce heat to medium low and cook until the vegetables are tender, about ten minutes.

2. Add corn and turkey and cook three or four minutes. (If using turkey cutlets, add with the corn and cook until just tender. If using cooked turkey, add a few minutes just before serving.)
3. Add lime juice and crushed red pepper. Season with salt and pepper. Serve with a dollop of sour cream, if desired. Serves four to six.

TURKEY CURRY

2 tablespoons canola oil
1 large onion, chopped
2 tablespoons all-purpose flour
1 and ½ teaspoons curry powder
1 (fourteen-ounce) can fat-free, less-sodium chicken broth
3 cups chopped, cooked turkey
Salt and black pepper to taste
2 tablespoons chopped fresh parsley or cilantro

4 servings brown rice
Mango chutney

Heat canola oil in a large nonstick skillet over medium-high heat. Add onion; sauté for four minutes. Add flour and curry powder; sauté for one minute. Stir in chicken broth; bring to a boil. Stir in turkey and salt and pepper. Reduce heat, and simmer several minutes until thickened.

Serve on cooked brown rice. Sprinkle with parsley or cilantro. Serve with mango chutney. Serves four.

I \'ī\(also i)
n. (pl. is or i's)
the ninth letter of the alphabet

IDAHO: PART ONE

Recipe: Baked Burritos

IDAHO: PART TWO

Recipe: Sourdough Starter

Recipe: Sourdough Bread or Rolls

Recipe: Sourdough Pancakes

IDAHO: PART ONE

We followed Lew, the Caldwell Farm Labor Camp manager, down the dusty, deep-rutted road in our overloaded Fairlane Ford until we came to House #3. "It's in better condition than most of the houses," he assured us as he unlocked the door.

I silently questioned those words as my eyes swept the kitchen cabinets, some with missing doors and oven door with no handle. It didn't take long to see the rest—four small rooms and a bath with shower only. A gigantic brown oil stove occupied a fourth of the space in the small living room. The sofa had holes. In the house just fifteen feet away, a record player blared with Latin music. Curious children and dogs suddenly appeared to hold open our door as we carried in our boxes and bags. Our little four-year-old Ann wandered into the backyard and got chased by the neighbor's rooster.

It was late in the afternoon after a week of travel, and I felt pretty depressed. "I just want a strawberry milkshake," I told Jay, so we drove back into the town of Caldwell, Idaho, to comfort our spirits with something sweet and creamy for supper.

Later that evening, we took our first walk around the camp and saw about forty houses similar to ours, each with two or three wrecked cars parked in back. Pretty, brown Mexican American children eyed us shyly as we passed and snatches of Spanish leaked out of loose fitting screen doors. In another part of the camp, we saw thirty-six cinder block row shelters intended to house six families each, one room per family. Common bath and toilet facilities were located in several central areas nearby. Huge trucks clattered over the potholes in the road, filled with tired, sweaty men and women returning home from twelve hours of farm labor in the fields of Canyon County.

After Ann and Jill were safely sleeping in their shared double bed, we looked at each other in disbelief and asked, "Why are we here?"

The answer to that question took us back to early 1968 after Jay had been granted a year of sabbatical leave from Eastern Mennonite High School. With the prospect of a new adventure, we contacted the Mennonite Board of Missions and Charities in Elkhart, Indiana, to explore the possibility of voluntary service. Eventually, we agreed on a placement with the Southern Idaho Migrant Ministry Committee of the Idaho Council of Churches.

A brochure from the National Council of Churches (1968) included a quotation from the U. S. Department of Labor. "'The migrant worker's year is a string of beads—a week of employment here, another there, uncertainty tied together with travel in search of work.' By the very nature of their work and lives, these migratory people are separated from the mainstream of society and rarely given the chance to lift their sights from the acres they work in search of a more humane existence." One of the National Council's goals at that time was to develop a program of Christian nurture with migrant people.

Without a specific work assignment, our directive seemed to be to learn to know the people in the camp and their needs so that we could relate those needs to the local Migrant Ministry Board who would in turn enlist support from member churches in the city of Caldwell.

Learn to know the people. In the peak season, the camp housed up to one thousand two hundred very transient people. In the forty houses where some families were more or less permanent, working in potato product industries during the winter months, three hundred more people lived. It was already late August, and the people in the row shelters would be returning to Texas border towns soon, so we decided to concentrate on the people in the houses.

A plan for connecting with a number of households came soon after we arrived. I took a plateful of warm home-baked cookies and went to visit a neighbor. Two little girls dropped in, sampled my cookies, and marveled that I had actually baked them myself. I realized that many of the little girls in the camp either had no oven or no one with time to bake cookies and teach them how. So began a stream of twenty-four cookie bakers between grades three and five, giving me contact with almost two dozen families. Many had never seen a flour sifter and were fascinated by my electric mixer. The twelve pairs baked twelve different kinds of cookies. Each little girl took home a dozen, and I kept about two dozen in the freezer of a community friend. Then one Sunday afternoon, we invited all the little girls and their mothers to a cookie party using the frozen cookies.

Several little girls stayed to help me clean up after the party. One touched my heart when she confided, "I like to wash dishes when the water is warm."

Actually, it wasn't hard to become acquainted with these naturally warm-hearted people. Previous volunteers had lived in their camp and earned their trust, so they welcomed us immediately as friends, not intruders. Within days, our dear neighbor across the street, Amelia Gonzales, brought roasting ears twice; and her husband, Adan, carried over a big bag of Idaho potatoes from the field where he had been working. Another family invited us to the birthday party of their one-year-old son, and we all took a swing at the piñata. The camp, in cooperation with the Migrant Ministry, held a fiesta in our honor with Spanish dances and a band of mariachi musicians. Mexican families love children, and our friendly little four-year-old twins provided the entrée into many conversations.

The second part of the job description, *learn to know their needs,* was not hard either. There were so many needs, and they were blatantly evident wherever one looked. The hard part was knowing what to do first and knowing that their poverty was so entrenched that there was very little we could do beyond the moment.

Many of the men had six months of unemployment during the winter months, and lack of purposeful activity led them to drink too much. Some families lacked clothes and food, rent money and medicine. There were mismanagement of resources, unwanted pregnancies, poor health, and no dental care. Programming for adults was very difficult, but education for the children and youth seemed more attainable. We were teachers, and we believed that education offered hope to the next generation.

One rainy morning in early November, I went to visit my new friend Vicky Menchaca. Her three little preschool boys were playing behind the stove, pounding blocks of fuel wood together and making a terrible racket. In the bedroom, one thin wall away, Grandma Menchaca, who had worked the night shift at a potato processing plant, was trying to sleep. Outside the four-room house, there was nothing but mud. Inside, there were no toys, no books, no games for rowdy preschool boys. Vicky was distraught, as any mother would have been, and told me in broken English, "Sometimes I cry. They will not listen to me. They cannot play outside."

Several weeks later, we began what we called the Play Care Project. Each Monday, Wednesday, and Friday morning, about twenty preschool children came to the Child Development Center (summer day care building) to play. Volunteers from Caldwell churches brought outgrown fire engines, trains, tinker toys, and dolls. For five months, we spent mornings reading books on the story rug, marching with paper hats and rhythm sticks, molding play dough, and doing paper crafts.

Perhaps we were dreamers, but if these children entered kindergarten with a better understanding of the English language, we would have been satisfied. If Grandma Menchaca got a few hours of uninterrupted sleep each day, and Vicky had some moments of peace and solitude, our dreams would have been more than fulfilled.

Most of the elementary school and teenage crowd had failed at least one grade, and there were serious problems with absenteeism and attrition. Students from College of Idaho and older teens from the churches were available for Saturday morning tutoring, and we helped with homework some evenings, even loaning our personal typewriter for practice, but many took only limited advantage of these opportunities.

Enrichment activities, such as the 4H Clubs, drew greater participation. Girls had lessons in cooking and grooming, while boys worked with wood and electricity. Senior highs from Boone Presbyterian Church came every Saturday morning for a recreational program that included special events like Kite Day and a snow adventure in the mountains of Bogus Basin. Women from the churches and I offered a weekly sewing class where teens made stuffed animals, pajamas, and other Christmas gifts. We outfitted bridesmaids for two large wedding parties, and a great many girls went happily to school wearing a new jumper or skirt. Teenage boys were organized to play basketball in the church league. Jay, who was taking theater classes at C of I, as requested by Eastern Mennonite College, turned his directing assignment into the successful production of "Once Upon a Playground" that was presented on the college stage as well as in the camp to an audience of over a hundred proud family members.

In May, after the seasonal farm workers returned from Texas, the Federal Office of Economic Opportunity made funds available for the operation of the day care center for children two and a half to six years of age. Children were brought as early as six o'clock in the morning and picked up again about twelve hours later when their mothers returned from the fields. They were fed a nutritious breakfast and lunch and given a program of education, rest, and recreation. I taught the five-year-old class, helped to serve lunches, and bent to rub backs until seventy-five to one hundred tired children were all asleep on their cots for an afternoon nap.

Our third directive was to *relate the needs to the Migrant Ministry Board so that they could enlist support from member churches*. Jay regularly attended the MMB meetings, and our family attended various churches, often two different ones on the same Sunday. This put us in contact with people in the city of Caldwell and gave us opportunities to inform them about the needs of their neighbors at the camp.

Churches of the Migrant Ministry—Boone Memorial Presbyterian, Faith Lutheran, First Methodist, Nampa Mennonite, Saint Mary's Catholic, Treasure Valley Christian, and others united to respond to the needs in the labor camp. They never let us down.

Boone Memorial Presbyterian gave extravagantly from their time and resources. Ruth Wendt came regularly to assist in the Play Care Program and in the Wednesday night sewing classes. When the public health nurse found two children from the row shelters whose skin was encrusted with scabs from impetigo, it was Ruth Wendt who graciously offered her gleaming white bathtub to soak and scrub them so medication could be applied. (People in the row shelters had no bathing facilities except showers with cold water.) Jim Moiso, associate pastor, brought the senior high youth group to camp every Saturday morning to lead a first-rate recreation program for upper elementary and youth. Sylvia Hunt, the church organist, gave free piano lessons to five little girls. Norma Nutting welcomed Fernando Molina, a little boy losing his eyesight from a congenital condition, into her home until other resources could be arranged. The church was also generous with material aid.

We found ourselves going back to Boone Sunday after Sunday. Not only did they meet camp needs, they met our needs as well, offering us friendship and spiritual renewal. Ruth and Bob Wendt remain our dear friends these many years.

Nampa Mennonite Church, a little distance away, felt like home. The pastor and his wife, Cleo, and Nellie Mann, an older couple, took us in and became like grandparents to Ann and Jill. The James and June Good family and the Archie and Erma Janzen family were our Christian brothers and sisters, and we often enjoyed their weekend hospitality.

Some of our dearest friends in Idaho lived right across the unpaved street from our House #3. They were Adan and Amelia Gonzales and their children—creative, introspective Adan Jr. (twelve); sweet and dependable Bertha (nine); and peppy, playful Diana (six). Our families ate together, played croquet in our back yard, occasionally went to a movie, and looked out for each other's children.

Amelia was a good cook and made delicious refried beans and rice. She cooked by heart, not by recipe. "Sometime, when you cook, let me come over and watch how you do it," I begged. I still have my notes from that visit in my recipe folder. Alas! I have never had the courage to attempt the intriguing procedures I witnessed that day!

Refried Beans
Cook pinto beans until soft. Season with salt and meat or meat drippings.

Fry beans in a skillet with lard. Mash with a potato masher as they fry, adding bean broth as needed to make a cream soup consistency.

Strain the "soup" through a sieve and fry the puree in another skillet until kind of dry.

Mexican Rice
Stew chicken gizzards and dice into small pieces.

Make a spice mixture by grinding two cloves of garlic, one teaspoon cumin powder, ½ teaspoon black pepper, and two cups canned tomatoes.

Fry one cup of rice in one-half cup of lard until the rice pops like corn.

Add chicken gizzards, one-half cup diced white onion, the tomato spice mixture, salt, and the broth from the gizzards.

Continue to fry until rice is soft and fluffy, adding more water, if necessary.

Less authentic but easy and delicious, Baked Burritos are reminiscent of the aromas and flavors we enjoyed among Mexican American cooks in the Caldwell, Idaho, Farm Labor Camp in 1968 and 1969.

BAKED BURRITOS

2 lbs. ground beef
2 fifteen-ounce cans low fat refried beans
1 envelope reduced-sodium taco seasoning
2 10 ¾ ounce cans cream of mushroom soup
2 cups reduced-fat sour cream
10 medium tortillas
1 and ½ cups grated cheddar cheese

Lettuce, cut into small pieces
Tomatoes, chopped
Salsa

1. Brown meat. Stir in beans and taco seasoning and set aside.
2. Mix together soup and sour cream. Pour half into greased nine-by-thirteen baking dish.
3. Spread a portion of the meat mixture into the center of each tortilla and roll up. Place filled tortillas in sauce in baking dish. Spread with remaining sauce.
4. Bake at 350 degrees for fifteen minutes. Sprinkle with cheese. Bake fifteen more minutes. Serve with lettuce, tomatoes, and salsa.

IDAHO: PART TWO

The little brown crock sat on the counter, a fermentation factory, bubbling slowly and sending its heady fragrance into our kitchen. At least once a week, we removed a portion of its contents to bake our bread and then "fed the starter" with another cup of flour and some lukewarm water.

Sourdough, which they say has been known since ancient times, was the main bread made on the American frontier as the search for gold and silver in the mid-1800s attracted thousands of miners to California, Colorado, Montana, and even Idaho. In those days, a sourdough starter was one of the most important possessions a prospector or a pioneer family could have, ranking right up there close to the Holy Bible. The starter was the wellspring of every meal used in making bread, biscuits, and flapjacks. It was kept alive and passed on from generation to generation. Mine was given to me by Jane after we made our second trek to Idaho. In some ways, our sourdough starter stands as the symbol of this two-year sojourn in the West.

We went back to Idaho in 1974 not in search of gold or silver but education. After five years of teaching at the college level, Jay felt a strong push in the direction of doctoral study. He searched for a program to his liking, a Doctor of Arts that focused on interdisciplinary teaching rather than on research, and discovered Idaho State University in Pocatello, Idaho.

Caldwell, where we had lived in 1968-1969, was located near the western border of the state where the Snake River leaves the Oregon line to cut across southwestern Idaho, watering the Treasure Valley. Pocatello is located in the southeastern part of the state close to Wyoming in the foothills of the Rocky Mountains along the Oregon Trail. Pocatello was founded as an important stop on the first railroad in Idaho during the gold rush. It was named after Chief Pocatello of the Shoshone Tribe who granted right-of-way for the railroad across the Fort Hall Indian Reservation.

Somehow, we learned about the Pocatello Heights apartment complex located about four blocks from the university and sent our two hundred-dollar deposit for a furnished two-bedroom unit. In late August, we pulled our U-Haul trailer into the paved driveway separating our building from its garages and unloaded the possessions we had considered essential, including my sewing machine. Apartment 3K was located on the first floor and at the corner of the building, giving us extra sunlight and easy access to the world outside our tiny space. It was clean and decent. I remember that the burnt orange carpet was still wet from a recent shampoo and a little squishy as we walked about on white paper strips to unpack our boxes.

The cupboard and refrigerator were empty, of course, so we drove around the unfamiliar city until we spotted an Albertson's Grocery where we found all we needed to stock our shelves. The first week was devoted to search and discovery as we oriented ourselves to our new home. We knew no one, and there was no fiesta in our honor as there had been in Caldwell!

Jill and Ann were rising fifth graders, sad to leave their Virginia home and friends but brave enough to make a good adjustment. Their new school was Greenacres, about two blocks from our apartment. When we went to preregister them, we met the principal, Dorothy Frazier, a stalwart woman with "competence" emblazoned across her large-boned frame. Her merry blue eyes sparkled as she talked with Ann and Jill and enrolled them into separate classes: Ann, with Mrs. Firkins; and Jill, with Mrs. Hill.

Mrs. Frazier's friendly interest in our family inspired our confidence, and we found ourselves telling her why we were in Pocatello. I revealed that, as a teacher, I had applied for a teaching job, even though I knew I was at a long-distance disadvantage. Before we left her office, she had offered me a job at Greenacres as a teacher's assistant. I was not assigned to a specific classroom but given a corrective reading group to teach using a classroom of my own, playground supervision, and office and library clerical work. Perfect! It was a job that would accommodate itself to Ann and Jill's needs, give me regular contact with people who could become my friends, and earn grocery money!

Jay began classes at Idaho State University and soon knew the other students in his program. Two had families and children. Byron Hill, his wife Earlene, and their children, John and Christie, were from Dodge City, Kansas. Jane Purtle and her children, Susan and Stephen, were from Batesville, Arkansas, where her husband John had remained with his law practice. We three families often shared meals, played games together, and even went on a weekend camping trip to Yellowstone.

Jane loved cooking and baking. The bread and rolls she served had a tangy flavor, light texture, and chewy crust. She had discovered sourdough and generously passed along a cup of her starter to us with several three-by-five cards on which she shared instructions and recipes. On one, she wrote, "I keep the starter in the refrigerator between times so that it doesn't get too sour. Take it out several hours in advance of using it so that it becomes active again. After using it, replenish the pot by adding flour and water to restore the mixture to its original amount and consistency. Let it work about a day (twelve to twenty-four hours) uncovered before storing it in the refrigerator again." Soon, Jay and I were baking our own bread on a weekly basis, loving the aroma as much as the loaf.

Sourdough, as a symbol of our two years in Pocatello, represents friendships and sharing with others. Sourdough must be used in order to remain active. Jane shared her starter, as well as the products of her baking, with us, and we were challenged to continue the gift with others.

Sourdough is a symbol of renewal and replenishment. Each time a cup is used for baking, it must be replenished with new flour and water in order to grow again for the next baking cycle.

The Pocatello United Methodist Church, conveniently located just across the street, met many of our needs for replenishment each week. On Monday, after our first visit to the church, two women dropped in to welcome us and left a loaf of bread. We were impressed with their outreach as we had been with their Sunday service and never looked further for a church. Actually, our choices were rather limited since about seventy-five percent of Pocatello's residents were Latter Day Saints (Mormon), and another ten percent were Catholic. There was no Mennonite church closer than Aberdeen, about forty miles away.

The United Methodist Church met our needs for weekly association with other Christians. Jill and Ann enjoyed their Sunday school class, and each Sunday as we made our way through the foyer to the sanctuary, they greeted the bust of John Wesley with a whispered, "Good morning, John!" Jay and the girls sang in choirs.

One night while they were all at choir practice and I was home alone, I heard a strange rumbling noise that quivered the apartment house. My first thought was "What in the world are the people upstairs doing?" and then I instinctively knew that I was experiencing an earthquake. I left the apartment and went into the parking area where others were coming from their apartments. We clustered on the pavement, sharing our thoughts and fears. (This was the only experience of community I witnessed among the apartment neighbors in the two years we lived there.) Later, we learned that the epicenter of the tremor was about seventy miles away—still strong enough to swing the chandeliers in the church, Jay reported.

Our Methodist friends invited us to their homes. Marge and Bill Brissenden invited us to join them for the weekend at their Salmon River mountain retreat, stopping along the way to see the Silver City ghost town. We joined a group for an evening at Lava Hot Springs where we bathed in the steaming waters while ice froze on the terrazzo surrounding the pools. Back in Virginia, we enjoyed visits from Ken and Vicki Light and family, Dorothy and Ivan Frazier, and Ron Hinson.

Sourdough can also be a symbol of challenge. Managing a starter requires careful attention to its needs. If neglected, it can push the lid off the crock and grow all over the counter top. If starved or allowed to get too hot, it will die. Our second year in Pocatello was a year of challenge for me.

In mid-August, my friend and mentor, Dorothy Frazier, learned that the school district had openings for two English teachers at the junior high level and encouraged me to apply. I was called for interviews at Hawthorne, a dirty downtown building with a rough reputation, and at Franklin, a new school in the suburbs of the city. I heard nothing for a few days and laid the prospect of an offer aside as our family eagerly anticipated the visit of my mother and two of her friends from Virginia.

We had a wonderful time with Mother, Frances, and Evelyn, showing them a bit of Idaho. As we were preparing for a weekend trip with them to Salt Lake City, a call came from Mr. Soderquist, principal of Franklin Junior High, offering me a job. Opening school conference for teachers was scheduled to begin the coming Monday morning, so I made a fast decision, signed a contract, and set out for Salt Lake City all in the same day.

There was no time to do long range planning for my five classes of seventh and ninth grade students, and I scrambled to stay at least a week ahead. Mr. Soderquist observed my teaching after several weeks and sent me a copy of his evaluation that was all marked "satisfactory" and included a strong statement of affirmation, "You are coming through loud and clear because of some excellent planning, the development of mutual respect, and the techniques that you use. From all that I see, we have added another excellent teacher to our staff. Well done! Now, how can we help you?" While I appreciated his confidence, it did not concur with my own evaluation. I knew that I was merely coping and not meeting my own standards for excellent teaching.

By October, the tensions concerning pay scale and working conditions between the teachers and the administration of Idaho School District No. 25 had reached the point of a strike. This posed a dilemma for me. I didn't want to be a scab and cross the picket line. Neither did I want to excuse myself from my fellow teachers' needs by saying, "I'll only be here for one year, so this doesn't affect me personally." In the end, I spent an afternoon with fellow teachers holding a placard at the entrance to our school yard. When I was urged to write a letter to the editor of the *Idaho State Journal*, they published my appeal to the newspaper "to be a part of the solution to this problem by not printing derogatory and recriminatory statements that are ill-founded in fact."

Although the percentage of African American people in the city was below the state average, racial tensions ran strong. One Monday morning when we teachers went to sign in, we viewed the man-sized hole in the cinder block wall where weekend vandals had broken into the school, using dynamite to enter the principal's office. I had a young man in one of my classes who had been transferred to Franklin because of serious misbehavior at another city school. Several schools in the city had gang members and drug users and found it necessary to remove all the doors from their restrooms. Many times I felt like discipline overtook education in the course of my day, and I went home exhausted.

I often felt homesick as my students worked on an assignment, and I looked out my classroom windows at the surrounding brown mountains of scrub brush beneath the winter sky. I missed the green and purple mountains of Virginia. One day, another teacher told me that he had hiked a part of the Appalachian Trail back East one summer. "I was never so sick of seeing *green* in my life," he concluded. Truly beauty is in the eye of the beholder!

As the year progressed, I had a revelation—I don't have to do this all of my life! Simple enough, but it shook my identity. I had never considered any employment other than teaching since I had adopted that goal way back in third grade. During the spring, I sent some inquiries and entered some negotiations which eventually led me to the Student Life Division at Eastern Mennonite College.

Fortunately, sourdough is also a strong symbol of survival! Self-styled connoisseurs of sourdough announce great claims for the longevity of their starters, some tracing back through three generations, claims Don Holm, author of *The Complete Sourdough Cookbook* (Caxton Printers, Ltd. 1974).

The Landis family survived our two years in Pocatello—and with gratitude for the overall positive experience. Jill and Ann flourished at Greenacres and came away with the rudiments for playing the cello and viola, instruments they continue to enjoy as adults. Jay persevered and earned his Doctor of Arts in English degree, undergirding the remaining thirty-one years of his teaching career. I was enriched by my wide variety of experiences, not the least of which was my association with two strong women, Jane Purtle and Dorothy Frazier. The solidarity of our family of four grew, often as we were nourished around our little table with slices of still-warm sourdough bread spread with butter and jam.

SOURDOUGH STARTER

Find a suitable container with a loose-fitting lid, such as a bean pot, butter crock, plastic bowl, or glass jar. (Never use a metal container.) Scald the bowl before use to inhibit the growth of unwanted bacteria.

Measure two cups of lukewarm water (nonchlorinated, if possible) into the container.

Sprinkle in one tablespoon of dry yeast and stir to dissolve.

Mix in two cups all-purpose flour (unbleached, if possible).

Stir to break up the lumps and let stand in a warm (not hot) place for at least twenty-four hours or until the pot gives off a delectable yeasty odor.

Cover the container but not tightly.

JANE'S SOURDOUGH BREAD OR ROLLS

Mix and let stand for fifteen minutes:
- 1 package dry yeast
- 1 tablespoon sugar
- ½ cup lukewarm water

Add:
- 2 teaspoons salt
- ⅓ cup oil
- ⅓ cup sugar
- 1 egg
- 1 cup lukewarm water
- 1 cup sourdough starter
- 3 cups flour

Additional 3 cups flour

Beat at low speed until smooth. Then add additional three cups flour. Stir well with spoon or hand. Turn out on floured surface and knead well for eight to ten minutes.

Rub oil in bottom of bowl and top of dough and set in warm place until double in size.

Punch down. Knead well again for several minutes. Shape into two loaves or two to three dozen rolls and put into baking pans.

Let rise again until double in size.

Bake rolls at 400 degrees about fifteen to twenty minutes and loaves at 350 degrees for forty to forty-five minutes. The loaf should sound hollow when tapped.

Makes three eight inch loaves or four dozen rolls.

SOURDOUGH PANCAKES

1 egg
1 tablespoon canola oil
½ cup buttermilk or low-fat milk
⅔ cup sourdough starter
½ teaspoon salt
1 tablespoon sugar
½ cup white whole wheat flour or all purpose flour
⅓ teaspoon soda and ⅔ teaspoon baking powder

Set the starter out of the refrigerator to warm to room temperature at least an hour before making the pancake batter. Beat the egg and oil in a large bowl.

Add milk, starter, salt, and sugar. Mix well. Combine the flour, soda, and baking powder. Slowly stir into the egg/milk mixture.

Bake over medium heat on a nonstick griddle that has been brushed with one teaspoon canola oil.

J

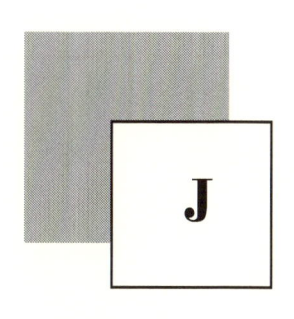

\'jā\ (also j)
n. (pl. js or j's)
the tenth letter of the alphabet

JIM

Recipe: Cracker Jack

JOURNALING

Recipe: Lentil Soup

JULIAN OF NORWICH

Recipe: Orange-Date Pumpkin Muffins

JIM

I remember a chilly morning in April 1943; I was three years and eight months old, and it is perhaps my earliest memory. The sun was not yet up when Daddy took me across the road to our neighbors, Miss Ella and her brother, Mr. Paul. Miss Ella settled me into Mr. Paul's little black coupe and put a couple of dresses from my brown bag "suitcase" across my legs to keep them warm before they drove me to Harrisonburg to meet my granddaddy at his feed store. Later, I learned that I had a little brother.

After several days, my grandparents took me home to meet baby James Dale (Jimmy) who was sleeping in blankets in my former crib. I asked to see his tiny feet and was told that I would have to wait until later when he woke up. Realization dawned that his convenience trumped my curiosity!

I did things to recapture center stage. I filled my mouth with water, puffed out my cheeks, and showed myself to Anna who had come to help Mother. Anna tapped my face, causing me to spew the water all over the floor in the hall, and then she insisted that I get a rag and wipe it up myself. One day when Jimmy was crying loudly, I suggested that we just flush him down the toilet, but no one liked that idea either!

As time went by, he became adorable, and I decided to lay claim on him. He was *my* baby brother! I fell quite naturally into the big sister role which requires one to assist the parents in "bringing up" a little brother. Usually, we were good playmates, well served by our imaginations. We were cowboys and owned large ranches, riding the heels off of our sumac stick horses. We converted old chicken houses into playhouses and made many delectable-looking pies from the mud we mixed. We played school, and I was his teacher. The neighborhood children were mostly girls, so he created an imaginary playmate named Harley who lived near the coal bin in our cellar. If we were going to town, Harley needed to be informed before we left.

We fought, of course. He was not about to take my bossiness without some resistance, and occasionally, his temper really flared. One of our tasks was to pump water from the cistern into the cows' watering trough. We traded turns at the pump, counting once at each revolution of the handle. One day when I counted faster than I pumped and an argument ensued, he picked up a rock and threatened to "kill" me. I could see that he meant to do it, so I ran, and he chased after me brandishing his rock until we were both exhausted and ready to settle it some other way.

During his high school days, I was quite proud of him. He was an outstanding athlete, good-looking with his "butch" haircut, and fastidious about his white buck shoes. He was fun and popular. I was not quite so proud of his academic performances, although he was a quick learner and could have brought home report cards that would have spared him Mother's constant scolding, "I *know* you could do better!"

He and his pretty childhood sweetheart, Ruby, married young, too young; they would agree. Within the next four years, my wonderful nephew and niece, Keith and Kim, were born, as were Ann and Jill. These four grandchildren had great fun playing together every Sunday afternoon when we all met at Grandma Heatwole's house on Chicago Avenue for food and family games. We played "Ducky, Ducky" when the kids were little and "Charades" when they grew older. One summer afternoon, we had a hilarious time acting out Bible stories in the backyard. Ann and Jill thought Uncle Jim was the funniest ham alive as he stomped through the lawn in his role of Goliath.

After high school graduation, Jim worked for Daddy on the farm for a year before taking a job with a small flooring business. Soon, he saw that he could do better in business for himself and began his journey economically upward as he moved from flooring to construction to real estate and property management. Along the way, he built new homes several times for his own family and sold them profitably before building another one.

In the 1980s, the economy took a dive, and Jim moved his business and eventually his family to the Washington DC area. He was not afraid of taking a business risk and was fortunate in his ventures. We were and are unalike in this respect. Never a brave adventurer, I have always worked for a salary and made conservative investments. As children, I nibbled my candy bar; he ate his!

In time, many things changed. Our children grew to adulthood and went their various ways. Jim and Ruby divorced. Living at a greater distance, we saw each other less frequently but still gathered for Christmas and significant occasions. Jim married Mary Elizabeth (Betty) Terry who is a charming addition to the family. Mother's health continued to decline, and she moved first to an assisted living facility and then to nursing care. More and more, our telephone conversations centered on Mother's care and her financial resources. Many times I consulted Jim about a problem situation and was always grateful for his wisdom and support.

In April 2008, the entire family, minus two busy great-grandchildren, gathered to celebrate Mother's ninetieth birthday. It was an entirely happy day. Jay and Ann went early to the Oak Lea Activity Room and arranged the tables with hydrangea paper ware, candles, and the four lavish flower arrangements Jim and Betty had sent. Our food was abundant with ham and lots of side dishes, fresh strawberries, Kim's famous homemade cookies, ice cream birthday cake, and more. Jim brought information from the Internet that compared prices in 1918 (the year of Mother's birth) with those in 1943 (his birth year), and he involved us all in a merry guessing game with his trivia questions. Everyone contributed to the gift certificate for Mother's beauty parlor visits. We relaxed around the tables and shared our stories about the wonderful times and delicious food we remembered at Grandma's house. Our greatest pleasure was seeing her so happy.

Three months later, in July of the same year, Mother died, and we all came together for a less happy occasion. Since then, members of the family have rendezvoused at various times and places but not as one. Sadly, we realize how much she was the magnet that drew us together.

Jim and Betty live in Naples, Florida, and Gainesville, Virginia. We meet for Christmas and for lunch in the summer, telephone occasionally, and remember birthdays. Friends and fortunes have taken us different ways, but family ties remain a strong bond that defies distance. Jim is no longer my baby brother but forever my favorite!

Mother loved to make "Cracker Jack" because she knew it was one of Jim's favorite snacks. Indeed, it is a fit finale for any family gathering!

CRACKER JACK

1 gallon popped corn

1 cup brown sugar
½ cup butter
¼ cup white corn syrup
¼ teaspoon soda

Combine brown sugar, butter, and corn syrup in a saucepan and cook at a slow boil for four minutes. Stir in soda.

Pour the mixture over the popcorn in a large bowl and stir to coat each kernel. Spread on two cookie sheets.

Bake in 200-degree oven for one hour.

Take from oven, and while still warm, break apart into snack-size clusters.

JOURNALING

I'm very grateful that I have a journal and that I can write because that helps me to objectify things that might just mess me around emotionally, otherwise. It gives them a pattern. A young poet went to Sidonie-Gabrielle Colette and complained that he was unhappy, and she said, "Who asked you to be happy? Write!" and I think that's very good advice. Journaling defuses things. It objectifies, and I can no longer look at this and weep and feel sorry for myself." Madeleine L'Engle, *The Life of Meaning*, Bob Abernethy and William Bole, editors, Seven Stories Press, 2007, p. 96.

Friday, January 1, 1999

Clean, new page! How awesome to begin to write in this book of 1999! This year and next (the turn of the millennium) are significant in ways I cannot even comprehend. To acknowledge the wonder of living at this time in history, I have decided to record some of my activities and thoughts over a two year period. These are the activities and thoughts of a white woman turning sixty years old this year, living in the United States, a Christian, employed by a financial institution of my church, married for thirty-seven years, mother, and grandmother.

This morning, I made lentil soup. Jay and I are on vacation, so we made it together, each preparing some of the ingredients for the pot that simmered slowly until the flavors merged into a rich blend of tomatoes, herbs, and legumes, kind of russet in color, full of vitamin C, and very sustaining on this cold day with temperatures below freezing.

I think it would be possible to draw a lot of parallels between the soup and my marriage that has usually been a cooperative venture and a most satisfying stronghold against all sorts of outside vicissitudes.

We took a pint to Mother for her supper—a kind of "giving back" for all the "warm soup" she has prepared for her family in her eighty-plus years.

Friday, December 31, 1999

It is now 12:23 a.m. and actually the New Year, Century, Millennium has begun as I write this!

To mark the event, Jay and I went to First Night in downtown Harrisonburg and spent the whole evening from 7:00 until after 12:00 o'clock. The exciting moment, of course, was when the crowd began to count down to 12:00 o'clock, and suddenly the fireworks took off—the most spectacular being fountains of white light all around the courthouse and spraying from the roof and porches too, plus some really beautiful ones in the sky show. Earlier, we heard comedy, theater, and music performances, met people we knew, drank hot chocolate and coffee, and attended a prayer service planned by the Interfaith Council.

The lights are still on everywhere, a good sign that Y2K (the computer system breakdown) will not deal the blow that some feared. Perhaps the preparations and nonperishable food everyone stored will just make us more ready for a winter storm or some such predictable event.

Earlier in the day, we worked hard cleaning the house, taking down the major Christmas decorations. Jill called this evening and said she and Craig are both feeling bad with sore throats; Tim has not let them sleep well for several nights, and the pink eye is still a problem. I will call in the morning and see if there is anything I can do to help.

My original plan of writing each day for Years 1999 and 2000 has extended until the present. Journal writing, as the last thing I do each day, has become a ritual. I put to bed the happenings of each day, often with a clearer understanding of their greater or lesser significance in the scheme of things. Then I put myself to bed. My journal will faithfully hold the record should I want to consult it—which I frequently do!

This hearty soup recipe makes a large amount—enough to share or serve for several meals or freeze for later. Wonderful and sustaining, served with hot cornbread and fresh fruit for dessert!

LENTIL SOUP

Combine in a five-quart soup pot
    1 lb. lentils, sorted and washed
    8 cups of water
Cook for thirty minutes on medium heat until lentils are tender. Add:
    4 carrots, sliced into thin rings
    2 stalks celery, diced
    1 cup chopped onions
    1 clove of garlic crushed
    46-ounce bottle low-sodium V-8 juice
    1 to 2 cups diced ham
    1 teaspoon dried oregano
    Dash of black pepper
Bring to a boil, reduce heat, and simmer until carrots are tender. Just before serving, add two tablespoons of red wine vinegar and one-half cup fresh parsley, chopped.

JULIAN OF NORWICH

It is this apprehension of the fullness of God's love which builds in Julian that remarkable assurance for which she is so well-known. When she says that "all shall be well, and all manner of thing shall be well," she is not just being optimistic; she is reflecting the certainty that God is in control however much we may feel from time to time that life is likely to overwhelm us. She herself knew suffering, both at the time of her revelations and in her subsequent life, but she is given confidence by the passion and compassion of Christ. Who Was Julian? Michael McLean, Julian Shrine Publications, Norwich, 1984, p. 16.

I caught my first glimpse of Julian in about 1990 when she was introduced by a college chapel speaker in the company of Henri Nouwen and Saint Francis of Assisi. The following Christmas, I put her writings on my wish list and was pleased to receive a copy of *Julian of Norwich: Showings* from Jill and Craig.

The book provided additional glimpses of the woman who wrote it in spite of her wish to remain hidden. When she wrote *The Revelations of Divine Love*, about six hundred years ago, she told readers to forget her and look at Jesus.

Julian of Norwich, mystic and writer (1342-1429), was a contemporary of Geoffrey Chaucer and the first woman to write a book in English. She wrote it over a twenty-year period while she was an anchoress living in a small room attached to Saint Julian's Church in the northeastern port city of Norwich, England.

On May 8, 1373, when Julian was thirty years old, God sent her an illness so severe that she was given the last rites of the holy church. The priest held a cross before her, instructing her to "look upon it and draw comfort from it." During the next twelve hours, she was given sixteen revelations of God's love. When she awoke and recovered from her illness, she wrote down what she had been taught, and today, her book is regarded as a spiritual classic throughout the world.

In November 1992, I had my third glimpse of Julian. Jay and I were with a cross-cultural student group and living in London. Our good friends, Erma and George Brunk, were spending a sabbatical semester in Cambridge. We took the train north to spend the weekend with them, and George rented a Vauxhall so we could go "touring." Our destination was Norwich, in search of whatever traces we could find of Julian in order to fulfill a long-time dream of mine.

In the city cathedral, we discovered a map for the half-mile walk to her small church and sanctuary. There, we visited the restoration of the tiny room where she had lived. Notable about this room were its three windows. One window opened into the church so that Julian could hear the services and receive the sacraments. Another window communicated with her servant's room by which she received human company and care. The third window opened into the courtyard so that she could give comfort and counseling to the burdened and perplexed of her day. Within the simple interior of this space, an unexplainable aura of peace surrounded us; it was as close as I will ever come to standing on "holy ground."

In June 2002, my close friend, colleague, and frequent confidant, Erma, died of colon cancer. Her family and friends were invited to share their memories and give tributes following a luncheon before the afternoon service at Lindale Mennonite Church. As I considered many stories I could tell, I remembered our visit to Norwich. The following words are from the tribute I spoke on that sad day.

As I have reflected during the last several days on this visit to Norwich and also on Erma's life, I have realized that Erma had three windows, very much like Julian's. Certainly, Erma had a window that opened into the church, and her faith was a significant part of her life. Through another window, she carried on her work and daily life in a practical, very organized way.

But it is through the third window that most of us here have known her best. This is the window through which Erma has offered comfort and counseling to us when we were "burdened and perplexed." Above all, Erma was our friend, a wonderful listener, a caring, compassionate sister.

It is with mixed feelings that I think of Erma today, perhaps even talking face to face with Julian herself because I know that Erma is experiencing a life that transcends time and place. In the fullest sense, she knows the truth of Julian's famous words. "All shall be well, and all shall be well, and all manner of thing shall be well."

What do we feed our friends when they are sick? What did her caregivers offer Julian when she, "Lay for three days and three nights, and on the fourth night, received all the rites of Holy Church and did not expect to live until day?" We do not know what herbal teas fourteenth century nurses brought their patients.

When Erma felt nausea after her chemotherapy treatments and wanted only bland foods, I took her my creamy rice pudding. Earlier when I was recovering from surgery, Erma brought orange-date pumpkin muffins, nutrient-rich with a wonderful intense flavor.

ORANGE-DATE PUMPKIN MUFFINS

1 cup all-purpose white flour
1 cup whole wheat flour
2 teaspoons baking powder
1 teaspoon soda
½ teaspoon salt
1 teaspoon ground cinnamon

1 large seedless orange, scrubbed and cut into 8 sections
1 large egg
1 large egg white
⅔ cup pumpkin puree
½ cup packed brown sugar
¼ cup honey or corn syrup
3 tablespoons canola oil

¾ cup chopped dates
3 tablespoons chopped walnuts or pecans

Preheat oven to 400 degrees. Line twelve muffin cups with paper liners or spray with nonstick cooking spray.

In a large bowl, whisk together flours, baking powder, baking soda, salt and cinnamon; set aside.

Place orange sections in a food processor and puree. Add egg, egg white, pumpkin, sugar, honey or corn syrup, and oil; process until mixed.

Make a well in the center of the dry ingredients and add the orange mixture and dates; stir with a rubber spatula just to moisten the dry ingredients. Spoon into the prepared muffin cups and sprinkle with nuts.

Bake for eighteen to twenty minutes or until the tops spring back when touched lightly.

Makes twelve muffins.

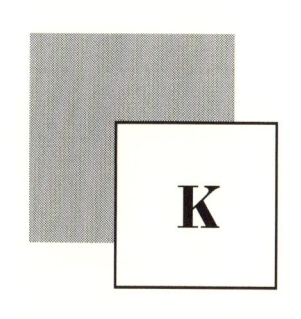

K \'kā\ (also k)
n. (pl. ks or k's)
the eleventh letter of the alphabet

KEEZLETOWN CHILDHOOD

Recipe: McIntosh Oatmeal Cookies

KEEZLETOWN CHILDHOOD

Heaven lies about us in our infancy;
Shades of the prison house begin to close
Upon the growing boy,
But he beholds the light, and whence it flows.
He sees it in his joy;
The youth, who daily farther from the east
Must travel, still is Nature's priest,
And by the vision splendid
Is on his way attended;
At length the man perceives it die away,
And fade into the light of common day.

In his poem "Ode: Imitations of Immortality from Recollections of Early Childhood," William Wordsworth (1770-1850) writes about his belief that children come from heaven "trailing clouds of glory." Later, he mourns the loss of childhood innocence, the loss of our connection to heaven.

This poem means more to me now in my seventies than it did when I first met it in high school. As I reflect on my childhood from this greater distance, I am surprised to find the pleasures so mixed with pain or fear in so many incidents. The joys of make-believe, birthday parties, double-dutch jump rope, hollyhock dolls, the walnut tree swing, and the horseback ride to the barn after their day of work in the field are offset by other darker memories of storms and fire, illness and death, mean animals, social isolation, loss, and the unfamiliar and unknown. To some extent, these brushes with the realities of the adult world are a predictable rite of passage, even an insurance policy against jumping headlong into dangerous circumstances.

Were the carefree days of childhood really carefree?

One summer afternoon, Mother slicked back my pigtails and told me to put on a fresh, clean dress before I went to my neighbor friend's house to play. Loretta was several years older, but we enjoyed blending our imaginations. On this hot afternoon, we took a pair of scissors and went into her back pasture to play "beauty shop." The field was frothy with an abundant crop of Queen Anne's Lace. One of us gathered several "ladies" and took them to the shop for a haircut. The "stylist" chopped off bangs on one edge and trimmed the rest either short or long as we chatted. For some of the "lacy ladies," it was "off with your head!"

We were so engrossed in our make-believe that we didn't notice the dark clouds until we heard thunder and felt the first big raindrops, so we ran for cover in a nearby abandoned chicken house to wait until the storm passed.

But it didn't pass! It grew darker and closer; lightning and thunder shook the old building, and the rain rolled down the windowpanes. What if lightning set the chicken house ablaze? Should we make a dash for Loretta's house? We pondered the possibilities in a rising panic. At last, Loretta made a decisive statement that put things into perspective. "If God wants us to die," she said, "then we will, but if God doesn't want us to die, then we won't." Somewhat comforted by predestination, we waited until the storm subsided. By then, our "ladies" had all drowned, and the beauty shop was flooded, so we took our scissors and went home, relieved that God had decided our fate in our favor!

Were the carefree days of childhood really carefree?

Our white bungalow stood on a grassy knoll three miles north of Keezletown where the sun came up late over the Massanutten Mountain. At the top of our hilly back pasture, a wooded area bordered the property line. Every day, Mr. Charlie came through the woods and walked down our hill to pick up his mail from the boxes at the end of our lane. Often, I walked back to the top of our hill with him and watched as he mounted the wooden stile over the fence and disappeared into the trees on his way home. He always walked with his hands clasped together at his back, so I did too, chattering all the way. I don't remember that he said much, but he seemed to enjoy my company.

One day, Mother heard that Ms. Dotsie, Mr. Charlie's wife, was very sick, so Mother prepared some food, and we climbed the hill to call. Ms. Dotsie was lying in her bed, asleep in a coma, with a large green ice cap on her head.

"She's dying," another neighbor whispered.

"If there's anything I can do to help, let me know," Mother whispered back in a neighborly way.

"Well," came the reply, "there's that dishpan of cucumbers. If you'd have time to can them into pickles, it'd be a big help."

So our afternoon took an unexpected turn! Mother was capable of handling such unforeseen circumstances, and she moved us into a process of washing the cucumbers in the cold waters of their spring house, slicing the pickles into jars, and cooking up a brine of salt and vinegar—all the time worrying that she didn't have a recipe, and they might not be very good!

A few days later, Ms. Dotsie did die, never to taste any of the pickles. I didn't know her very well, but I thought about her lying there in bed in her green ice cap and felt sorry for my friend, Mr. Charlie.

Were the carefree days of childhood really carefree?

When Daisy freshened and the calf needed her milk, we bought our milk from Mrs. Royer.

Mother had made Jimmy a winter overcoat from an old one belonging to Daddy. Jimmy's small version of the brown tweed had two huge patch pockets covering his rib cages, each big enough to carry a quart jar. So we set off on the bicycle to get milk: I, peddling; and he, riding behind on the seat with the jars in his pockets. We were terrified to ride past Mr. Ed's pasture where his mean bull sometimes bellowed and pawed the earth and grateful when he was not in sight. We watched as Mrs. Royer filled the glass jars with milk and tucked them back into Jimmy's pockets.

Peddling home again, my legs felt incredibly tired. I knew why, of course. Surely I was coming down with polio. In those days before the Salk vaccine, infantile paralysis was every parent's grave concern, and children were quick to sense their fears. I felt sure this would be my last trip to get milk, but fortunately, I was wrong. After a little rest, I was once again granted a reprieve.

Were the carefree days of childhood really carefree?

Susan and Nellie lived in an austere brick house near ours. They were the neighborhood children closest in age to me and Jimmy, and we spent hours playing "house" on the rock bluff, exploring the woods, making mud pies, and jumping rope. Theirs was a three-generation family, and they lived in their elderly grandmother's house. Their uncle, who had a well drilling rig, frequently visited his mother. One day when I was playing with Susan and Nellie, he invited me to come and sit on his lap. Little alarm bells went off inside my head! Why did this man who had never paid any attention to me before want me to sit on his lap? I said no; I had to go home. After that, I never went to their house when I saw his truck parked out front.

Were the carefree days of childhood really carefree?

When I was six, the yellow bus began to stop at my lane, and I joined the other neighborhood children for the ride to Keezletown High School, a grade one to twelve school serving about three hundred students. I was intimidated by the high school boys who sometimes teased me and Cleo, another first grader who occasionally sat beside me on the bus. Little innocents, we hadn't yet learned that boys and girls can't be friends.

The school house was a huge two-story brick building on a hill. It was necessary to climb two flights of concrete steps, more than a dozen in each flight, to enter the front door. Inside, first graders walked past the long oiled wooden stairs to the second floor and past the door that led to the darkly mysterious underworld from which the janitor emerged from time to time. To the right was our sunny classroom where Miss Earman gathered us under her grandmotherly wings. She was a rather plump, rosy-cheeked lady who wore an enormous knot of beautiful white hair high on her head.

Miss Earman issued each of her first graders a Dick and Jane reader, arithmetic workbook, and a coarse blue-lined writing paper tablet. But the supply article, I remember best was the pencil. It was dark blue with a narrow orange line on each of its eight ribs.

Periodically, Miss Earman's lesson plans called for a resharpening of the pencils. Then row by row, she called us to the pencil sharpener for a fresh point. Some little boys were delighted with the mechanical wonder known as the pencil sharpener and ground away with abandon. But I always heard in Miss Earman's instructions a clear call to conservation, so much so that I sometimes did not even go to the sharpener when my row was called. Then one day, Miss Earman decided to make a moral lesson of me and my pencil. She held it up, displaying its full length of seven inches. By contrast, she held up some little boy's grubby stub, barely an inch and a half above the eraser. The attention embarrassed me a little then and even more today. I was the little girl who was so conscientious about the rules that she often wrote her lessons with a dull point!

A few weeks into the school year, I felt sick at school and was taken to a small room with a cot where I lay to wait for my parents to come for me. At home, I soon felt a little better and was able to play in the yard with Pal, our dog, and even turn a few somersaults in the grass. The next day when I felt sick again, no one came to take me home.

Being from perhaps the only Mennonite family in the school, I sometimes sensed a difference between my classmates and me. I was the only girl in my class with pigtails. Every morning, my mother braided my thick hair into French braids and tied the ends with ribbons that matched my dress. Once when the teacher used two toothpicks to check everyone's head for lice, she said, "I'm sure you don't have lice because your mother takes good care of your hair!"

The school bus took a long circuitous route home each day to discharge its load of pupils. One afternoon, we passed a house that had completely burned to the ground that day; smoke still wafted upward from the charred timbers. Somebody said that a little child sleeping upstairs had lost his life. On subsequent days, I turned my head and looked out the opposite window as we passed.

Other days, the bus ride home from school was fun! Our kind old driver was Mr. Hezekiah Huffman. As we neared a certain dip in the road which sometimes lifted our bottoms from the seats, we would grab the rail on the seat ahead and yell, "Hezzie, do a hundred!" Often, he speeded up a little to give us our momentary thrill. Occasionally, Hezzie stopped at a service station for gas and allowed the kids to get off the bus and buy ice cream. Once when I didn't have a dime for ice cream, he gave me one. No wonder I remember him so fondly!

Were the carefree days of childhood really carefree? As I grew older, my "clouds of glory" continued to evaporate, and I lost more and more of my early childhood innocence.

But when the clouds are gone, what does one have but sunshine! Most days were sunny. My home was a safe haven. When I scampered up the driveway and threw my book bag in a corner, Mother was there to welcome me. Often, the kitchen smelled like freshly baked cookies.

Here is Mother's old recipe for McIntosh Oatmeal Cookies, so sustaining with a glass of milk!

MCINTOSH OATMEAL COOKIES

1 cup sugar
1 cup butter, softened
1 and ½ cups of flour
1 teaspoon soda
1 teaspoon cinnamon
½ teaspoon salt
1 teaspoon vanilla
2 large eggs
2 medium McIntosh apples, peeled, cored, and diced
3 cups quick-cooking oatmeal
1 cup raisins
1 cup walnuts, chopped

Cream the butter and sugar. Add eggs and vanilla and beat until light and fluffy.

Sift flour, soda, cinnamon, and salt. Add to the creamed ingredients and mix well.

Stir apples, oats, raisins, and walnuts into the dough by hand.

Drop by rounded teaspoons onto a lightly oiled or nonstick cookie sheet.

Bake at 350 degrees for approximately twelve minutes.

Makes four and a half dozen cookies.

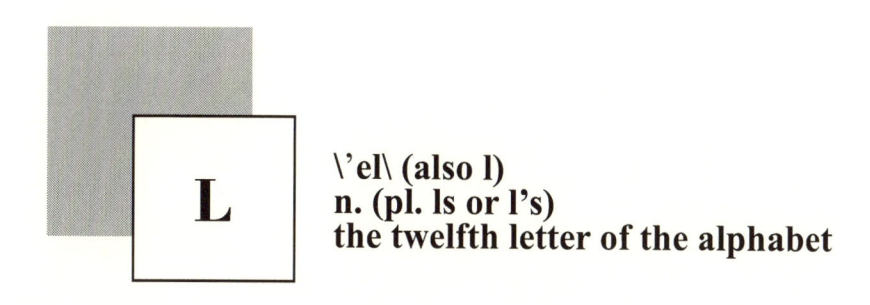

L \'el\ (also l)
n. (pl. ls or l's)
the twelfth letter of the alphabet

LANDIS AND GOOD FAMILIES

Recipe: My Chicken Corn Soup

LANDIS AND GOOD FAMILIES

I am an "in-law"—a relative by marriage. I have hundreds of these relatives, mostly in Pennsylvania, a set of characters that reads like the "L" and "G" sections of a telephone directory or the personae of a weighty Russian tome.

A careful genealogist could trace the Landis lineage by some very circuitous path all the way back to Hans Landis who lived in the canton of Zurich, Switzerland, an Anabaptist preacher who lost his life for his faith on September 29, 1614, in his seventieth year. Hans, the last Swiss martyr, was beheaded because he would not promise to cease his preaching. After the execution, the Zurich council decided to confiscate Anabaptist property without respite, forcing the family to leave the country. Some settled in the Alsace and later the Palatinate. About 1717, brothers Benjamin, Felix, and John Landis immigrated to Pennsylvania. Benjamin, a preacher, went to Lancaster. His lineal descendants are numerous, and many live in Lancaster County.

More than a hundred years later, Jay's great-grandfather, also a Benjamin Landis (1848-1916), and great-grandmother Lydia Catherine Zimmerman (1859-1934) had a family of ten living children. The litany of their names, "Jake and Ike and Ben and Mart and Alice and Phares and Cora, and Harry and Martha and Elmer," is the rhythmic chant so often repeated by Jay as he remembers his grandfather Martin's family. This generation produced twenty-nine offspring, and I have met many at Landis family reunions.

These great aunts and uncles and their families were well-known to Jay because his grandparents, Martin I. (1887-1962) and Emma Jane (Sheaffer) (1887-1962), lived with Jay's family. Their siblings visited often, and Jay's father's youngest cousins were Jay's playmates. Jay's father was an only child, and Jay had no closer Landis cousins.

The home of Samuel B. Good (1879-1970) and his wife Lillian W. Loose (1886-1965) stood on Front Street in the Moravian town of Lititz, an eleven-mile drive north of Lancaster City by horse and surrey or by touring car. Samuel, Jay's maternal grandfather, was the son of a Mennonite preacher, but being a bit of a renegade in his youth, he did not join his father's church and married Lillian in 1904, a stylish young lady from the Reformed tradition.

By 1915 when the Good family was well on its way, Preacher Sanford Landis from Mellinger's Mennonite Church held meetings in the area, following which Samuel and Lillian were baptized and became lifelong members of Lititz Mennonite Church. Samuel worked hard for the railroad and trap factory, and Lillian very successfully managed the account book and the family. Their lively fun-loving progeny of ten included Erla, Beulah,

Elwood, Esther (Jay's mother), John Henry, Howard, Wilmer, Richard, Naomi, and Elmer, their spouses, and seventeen grandchildren.

Though distant, these people are important to me because they are important to Jay and because they are my daughters' very own flesh and blood. In truth, they are not so much my in-laws, as I am the in-law, the adopted member into these friendly families.

The catalog of names, vague pictures of faces infrequently met, voices tinted with Pennsylvania Dutch tones, and family trees mysteriously intertwined swim together in the sea of my memory. Over the years, some have come ashore as significant individuals. I was fortunate to meet all four of Jay's grandparents.

The Landis and Good families joined hands when Martin Sheaffer Landis (1911-1993) and Esther Mae Good (1910-1987) said "I do" on January 1, 1931, in the home of Bishop Noah Landis.

Martin S. and Esther began housekeeping and farming on his father's farm, a thirty-acre tract on Route 896—the road that links Smoketown to the Lincoln Highway. Martin's parents, Martin I. and Emma, continued to live on the farm, but Martin I. began employment with his brothers Ben and Elmer at Landis Brothers Farm Equipment Company. A year and a half later, Jay was born on September 20, 1932, the day following his grandmother's birthday. In 1936, Jay's sister Marlene joined the family; and in 1942, the third Martin Landis arrived.

By the time I came into the picture, Jay was living and teaching in Virginia, and the parents and grandparents had moved into two separate houses on a poultry farm on Millport Road. The person I remember most from my first visit was Grandma Emma. She had lost her leg to cancer in her early forties and wore a prosthesis, but nothing stopped her. A member of the Reformed denomination before her marriage to a Mennonite, she somewhat resented the plain clothing that allowed no jewelry. As a last vestige of style, she pinned on her prayer covering with colored pins that matched her dress! Her brown eyes glowed with warmth as she showed me the gifts recently received at their golden wedding anniversary celebration, and they snapped with awe and intensity as she described yesterday's "wonderful wreck" on the Old Philadelphia Pike. ("Full of wonder" was a usage not found in my Shenandoah Valley-based vocabulary.)

Very generous people, Jay's grandparents and parents gave me an early wedding gift of a Model 401-A Singer sewing machine that I have loved to use (and used with love) all these years. I sewed my own wedding dress and daughter Jill's with that dependable friend.

The grandparents loaned us their rather new Corvair for our honeymoon. Sadly, that same car spun out of control on a wet highway one rainy night the following summer when Grandpa was blinded by the lights of a semi approaching over a hill. Before seatbelts were standard equipment, both grandparents were thrown from the car and lost their lives in August 1962.

So many gifts have come our way from our Pennsylvania family. Two weeks after our wedding, I put on my gown again to attend the dinner reception hosted by Mother and Daddy Landis at a Denver, Pennsylvania, restaurant. All the aunts and uncles, cousins and friends came, bearing gifts to bless us on our way. Grandma Good gave us twelve hand-crocheted lace doilies, the kind she would have used to dress the arms and backs of her parlor chairs. (I have never used them, but I treasure them in my chest. Also sheltered there is the too-pretty-to-use quilted blanket given by Uncle Abe and Aunt Fannie Sheaffer.) Sheets and pillow cases, towels and trays, pitchers and glasses stocked our shelves. We remember these givers when we use Aunt Hilda's salad bowl, cousin Glen's butter dish, and little nephews Robin and Dale's wooden rolling pin.

Mother and Daddy visited us in Virginia while I was still a nervous new bride. "Peggy, come here!" Daddy called me to the kitchen in what I thought was a rather brusque, commanding voice. "What have I done?" I wondered, only to find that he had gone to town and bought me a gift—a sturdy food grinder that clamped to the table, capable of grinding meat or the fresh cranberries I needed for my salad! He always brought his tools and did all the fix-it jobs we had on our list. On many trips, Mother and Daddy unloaded a chest of freshly dressed chickens and frozen vegetables from their garden straight into our freezer.

Jill and Ann loved to visit their grandparents in Pennsylvania, especially when there were baby chicks in the broiler house. Grandma played board games and laughed at their antics. Grandpa fried all the bacon they could eat for breakfast. (We rationed them to two strips each!) On holidays, Mother roasted a turkey—the best I've ever eaten—tender and juicy with hints of the celery and other vegetables she laid in the cavity. I try to do it like she did, but mine is never as good. Every New Year's Day, Daddy fried oysters that became a family tradition.

They moved at a faster pace than I did, south of the Mason-Dixon Line. Daddy drove faster, ate faster, hustled from dawn to dark. Food consumed a major part of Mother's day—gardening, preserving, cooking—before she dashed off to a church meeting with Daddy. He officially retired twice—once from pastor and once from superintendent at a church camp—then continued to work part-time as a visitation minister. When they retired the first time, the youth group gave them each a pair of roller skates!

At age seventy-seven, Mother gave me a gift I was reluctant to receive. She was lying in bed, suffering from Lou Gehrig's disease, when she asked me to find her sewing basket and offered me her silver thimble for my collection. "Oh, no," I declined, "you might need it." We both knew she was dying, but

I was in denial. She passed away a few months later in a Lancaster hospital, a day after our last visit to her in October 1987.

Later, Daddy married Nell Snyder, a widow in his Sunday school class. They lived together happily for four years near Oxford, Pennsylvania, until his death from stomach cancer in August 1993.

Our little branch of the Landis-Good family moves on—under different names and in settings far from its Lancaster County origin. Rebecca Snider was born to Jill and Craig in Meridian, Mississippi, eight days after Daddy's death. She was followed by little brothers, Nate in 1996, and Tim in 1999, both born in Florida. Ann moved to Florida in 1994, and Jill's family moved back to Virginia in 1999.

"We must remind them of their Pennsylvania heritage," we agreed, and so we planned a family weekend in May 2003.

To take the children back to Grandpa Jay's boyhood, we chose a farm stay. Meadow View K Farm Guest House was semidetached from the main house with a big kitchen and plenty of family room and bedroom space. Located near Mount Joy, the farm delivered all the brochure promised—baby kittens, a funny-eared rabbit, Dalmatian dog, chickens that laid eggs, and lots of calves and cows—plus a welcome from the congenial owners, Barry and Sharon Kreider.

I took food for our Friday evening meal around the big oval table. Timmy, who turned four that weekend, offered to say a "farm prayer" that went on at some length as he remembered cows and grass and other life so abundant in that Garden Spot of Pennsylvania Dutch Country. After supper, we played an "Ask Grandpa" game that gave Jay an opportunity to tell stories about his boyhood. Who was his dog, and why did he once spell "yellow" with three "Ls," we questioned.

Saturday was a full day of touring. We began with downtown Lancaster's Central Market where the bounty of the fertile earth is displayed in arrays of fresh vegetables, rings of sausage, wedges of cheese, homemade donuts, soft pretzels with mustard, cans of chow-chow, and everything else so enticing. Then we began our driving tour of Jay's landmark places: Locust Grove Elementary School, Lancaster Mennonite High School, the farm on Route 896, Mellinger's Church where Jay was baptized and where his grandparents are buried, the Good family home on Front Street in Lititz, not far from the Pretzel Factory. Midafternoon, we paid a short visit to the Landis Valley Museum, a nationally significant living history museum that interprets nineteenth century Pennsylvania German culture.

In the evening, we met siblings and their families at the Country Table Restaurant in Mount Joy. Jay's sister Marlene was there with husband Bob Shepard; their son Robin and wife Dawn; and Dale's son Michael; (absent: Dale, Judy, Nancy, and families) Jay's brother Marty and wife Ruth; their son Bryce, wife Kim, and son Evan; son Brian; daughter Beverly and husband Mark Thompson (absent: Wendell and family, Brian's family). These, plus our eight, made up the largest reunion of the family since Daddy's death in 1993.

On Sunday morning, we celebrated Timmy's fourth birthday! After the gifts were opened, we gathered around our country kitchen table to watch him blow out the candles on his sticky bun cake and to enjoy the farm-fresh strawberries bought the morning before at Central Market.

Our last stop was around the gravestone of Martin S. and Esther M. Landis in the village cemetery in Oxford, Pennsylvania. There, we sang a hymn together, read a psalm, and laid flowers—our hearts grateful for their love and for the heritage they had bequeathed to us.

When anyone says "Pennsylvania Dutch food," my mind goes immediately to Chicken Corn Soup of which there are many versions and nuances; some use potatoes instead of noodles; some add hard boiled eggs. Here is the version of a Shenandoah Valley "in-law!"

MY CHICKEN CORN SOUP

1 small onion, chopped
2 stems celery, chopped
2 carrots cut into thin rounds
6 cups low-sodium chicken broth

2 cups cooked chicken, chopped
2 cups fresh or frozen corn
½ teaspoon salt
¼ teaspoon black pepper

2 cups egg noodles, cooked according to package directions and drained

2 tablespoons fresh parsley, chopped
6 slices bacon, fried, drained, and crumbled

Simmer onion, celery, and carrots in chicken broth until tender, about fifteen minutes

Add chicken, corn, and seasonings. Return liquid to a gentle boil.

Add cooked noodles and more broth or water to make desired consistency.

Just before serving, add chopped parsley. Garnish with crumbled bacon. Serves six.

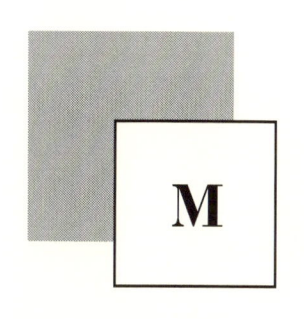

M \'em\ (also m)
n. (pl. ms or m's)
the thirteenth letter of the alphabet

MOTHER: HER LATER YEARS

Recipe: Pink Baked Apples

MOTHER: HER LATER YEARS

"Your mother is so sweet!"

How many times did I hear that adjective used to describe my mother? I agreed, of course. I didn't suggest that her personality may have been somewhat influenced by preparing and partaking of so many sweet desserts throughout her life—sour cream coconut cake, apple dumplings, butterscotch chip cookies, snow pudding with raspberry sauce, white Christmas pie, chocolate pecan turtles. In her file, "sweet" recipes surpassed all other categories combined, two to one!

Life itself was not always sweet, however, and served her two bitter platters.

When Mother was at her life's midpoint, age forty-five, she left the farm and moved into a small apartment, a single woman in a church culture that did not sanction separation or divorce. She acted with counsel from her pastor and doctor, removing herself from an irreconcilable situation. She had the support of her children and the friends who knew her best. More than once, I heard her say she believed it would be easier to be a widow than single because of separation.

Her second bitter platter was a neurological condition that developed sometime later and resulted in a continual weakening of her legs so that walking became gradually more and more difficult. Extensive testing did not entirely reveal the cause, but the doctor ultimately declared it an unusual strain of multiple sclerosis.

These problems forced her into greater dependency on her family. When she left the farm, she had never driven anything but a tractor. Uncle Harold, her brother mechanic, found her a used not-quite-red, not-quite-pink Plymouth, a color she called "tomato soup." Jay and I spent evening hours on the back roads north of Harrisonburg teaching her to signal, brake, and park before she went for her license.

Her first public job was in food service at Virginia Mennonite Home. She brought all the skills of food preparation she needed and soon discovered new skills when she became the manager there.

With money she inherited and her own careful management, she was able to purchase her first home, a neat little brick house on Chicago Avenue. To earn a bit extra and to fill lonely evenings, she began a second job as evening clerk at a small locally owned motel. Early one afternoon, a man came to the desk and asked to engage a room. Mother was uncertain which rooms had been cleaned and made ready for use, so she left briefly to talk to the housekeeper. When she returned, the man had the cash drawer open and his hand in the till. He looked at Mother, and she looked at him. Quietly but firmly, she said, "Put the money back into the drawer and close it, or I will call the police." What was there about this plump, petite, soft-spoken woman that moved him to close the drawer and beg her pardon with tears in his eyes, saying, "I never did that before, and I'll never do it again"?

Her children and grandchildren gathered almost every Sunday afternoon at the little Chicago Avenue house. She always fed us—if not a big dinner of baked steak and mashed potatoes, then a delightful supper of sandwiches, deviled eggs, and apple pie. The whole group played games together, or the grandchildren got out her toy box and built a tower of plastic stacking rings as high as the staircase or played "King of the Mountain" on the little hill in the front yard.

When climbing the stairs to her bedroom became more difficult, she sold the little brick house and bought a convenient one-story in Park View, just several blocks from our home and her new food service job at Eastern Mennonite College. An apartment in the basement provided income, often from itinerant college students. They brought along their loud music, motorcycles, and other simple or serious problems. Within a few months, through cookies and attentive listening, she tamed the wild ones into friends. They tried out their ideas on her, taught her about other cultures, and brought their parents to visit. Some may have added grey hairs, but they also kept her young at heart. We used to tell her she should write a book!

Work and people were antidotes for lonely evenings and weekends. She was part of a friendship quartet, two Hazels and a Reba, who shared their favorite foods with each other every Sunday after church and then played Scrabble well into the afternoon. They laughed themselves silly, remembering old stories like the time young Mother and one of the Hazels were riding a mule. They came upon Minnie Whitmore carrying her suitcase and decided to be good little Samaritans. When they lifted the suitcase on board, it spooked the mule, and he dashed off, leaving them no alternative but to throw Minnie's suitcase into a ditch!

Like the proverbial wise woman who "made coverings for her bed," so did Mother—and not just her bed but her daughter's beds, her granddaughters' beds, her seven great-grandchildren's beds, her friends' beds, and relief sale beds. Quilting was a lifelong pleasure she learned from her mother. When the minister at her funeral spoke of the saints in white robes around the throne, Granddaughter-in-law Dawn observed that hers would be a quilted one!

As her eightieth birthday approached, the family began to plan for a luncheon to honor the occasion. She demurred, not liking attention focused on her, but we persisted. Family and friends, nieces, nephews, and neighbors came together for a beautiful luncheon in Park View's social hall where ten round tables were set with pink cloths and potted geraniums. Jill and Ann constructed paper quilt squares, and guests were invited to sign colorful pieces to be glued into each square. The resulting book was hers to treasure, full of tributes such as:

- Thanks so much for all the good years and wonderful influence you have been on my life. You truly are a one-of-a-kind mother! Love, Jim (son)
- No matter what time of the day or what day of the week, I have *always* felt welcomed into your home! You always have time to talk and to listen—and express a genuine interest in our family . . . Thanks! Linda (neighbor)
- I remember as a child visiting in your home. The food was so delicious, and you were such a kind, loving person. I remember you with love! Shirley (niece)
- At Grandma Dot's: candy dish, ring-a-majigs, pizza, and sweeping with the little broom. I love you, Nate (great-grandson)
- You have been a true friend to our family and a real inspiration to me. I especially enjoy laughing with you at WMSC or wherever we are together. We can be serious, and those times are meaningful too. Love you, Ruth (friend)

Over the years, Mother's health and mobility continued to decline, although her mind remained clear until the end. She took expensive medicine to ease the pain in her arthritic knees. She went from her cane to a walker and ultimately to a wheel chair. She lost interest in her bank account, and Jay took over her checkbook, paying the monthly bills. I took her to doctor appointments and weekly hair appointments and did her grocery shopping. Frequently, I cooked enough to make a plate for her too and rushed it down the hill at suppertime.

Pleasant and jolly with friends, she was sometimes despondent with me. I read from her words and implications that she expected me to *do something* to solve her problems—to fix things. When I tried, it was often wrong. Once she told me how badly she wanted some new shoes and how hard it was to shop, so I decided to give her a pair for a birthday present. I went to the shoe store, selected about six pairs in a variety of styles and colors, charged the whole batch, and took them to her to choose which she liked best. I could tell immediately, almost before she saw them, that she wasn't going to like any of them. I offered to take them all back and try again, but she rather petulantly decided to keep one pair. So much for trying to fix things! I was not prepared for her disapproval. Was the problem that she was really mourning her loss of shopping, or did I do something wrong?

I found the switch of Mother-Child roles hard to accept. Understanding her right to feel helpless in her situation, I still resented the cheerful face she presented other visitors so soon after scolding me for not coming sooner or oftener. She resisted the thought of leaving her house, but I could not find myself willing or able to give my days and nights to nursing care.

> "What trick of motherhood is this
> Which overwhelms a child with guilt
> And makes her offspring feel remiss?"

wrote Geraldine Craig in a poem which spoke to some of the ambivalence I felt.

The tipping point came in the year 2000 when Mother could not follow the lines on the baby quilt she was stitching. She was admitted to the hospital with a slight stroke and released to a nursing care facility for six weeks of therapy. She returned home, and with assistance from a home health service, several housekeepers, and us, she managed for several months. When a call came saying that there was a room available in Crestwood, the assisted living facility at Virginia Mennonite Retirement Center, she acknowledged her need and reluctantly agreed to go. On the day following her admission, we took care of the perishables in her refrigerator. I felt tears as I poured the last of her iced tea from the stained Tupperware pitcher down the drain.

For three years, Mother motored around Crestwood at "turtle speed" on the scooter Jim bought her. We bought her a small quilting frame, and she made baby quilts for relief. Her Bible study group from church met weekly in her room, and she served them the cookies I brought her for the occasion. We often joined her in watching the cooking channel on TV, something she enjoyed for the rest of her life. Her chief complaint was that they didn't scrape their bowls clean enough!

In August 2003, Mother fell when transferring from bed to wheel chair, an event that precipitated a series of hospital visits and a permanent move to nursing care. "I hope I never have to go to Oak Lea," Mother often had said as she anticipated the future. But when she was settled into her room, she relaxed into the gentle care of the nursing staff, and I never heard that statement again. Always polite and gracious, she thanked the aides for every pitcher of iced water they brought during the next five years.

On the eve of Mother's ninetieth birthday, her whole family gathered in the Activity Room, made beautiful with a large table set for all and decorated with four floral arrangements sent by Jim and Betty. I took baked ham, scalloped potatoes, broccoli salad, and a bowl of fresh strawberries. Dawn and Jill added more salads, and Kim supplied three kinds of her famous home-baked cookies to complement the ice cream birthday cake. After the meal, we stayed at the table to share our memories, many of them involving mouth-watering foods Mother had served. Ann, Jill, Keith, and Kim kept us laughing with stories of things they did as children at Grandma's house. When we wheeled Mother back to her room, we found another forty birthday cards left by the mailman. Seeing Mother so happy that day made us so happy too.

Memories of that special day supported us three months later as she lay for nine days in her hospital bed, her condition worsening from pneumonia with sepsis, until death took her early on July 9, 2008. Two days later, we said goodbye in Weaver's Cemetery as each family member placed garden flowers—hydrangeas and daisies—on her casket. Her faithful pastor, Mark Keller, spoke from Psalm 23 and Revelation 7, declaring that we could have the sure knowledge that she is dwelling in the house of the Lord forever. (Dorothy Frances Suter Heatwole, 1918-2008)

We invited everyone present at the service, maybe a hundred and fifty people, to the luncheon that followed in the church social hall. Mother would have wanted that. She was known for her warm hospitality and loved nothing more than feeding her family and friends.

Pink Baked Apples was one of Mother's "sweet" recipes that I love to serve. I called her on the telephone shortly after my marriage to ask how to make them. She gave me the ingredients and instructions from memory, and I made notes on a scrap of paper, now much stained, that is still in my recipe file. Here is a more carefully written version:

PINK BAKED APPLES

6 to 8 medium baking apples, peeled, and halved. (Remove core with melon ball maker.)

1 tablespoon cornstarch
½ to ¾ cup of sugar, depending on tartness of the apples
1 cup boiling water
Several drops red food coloring
1 teaspoon vanilla

Nutmeg, walnuts, marshmallows
Arrange apples in a shallow baking dish, sprayed with cooking spray.
Put walnuts into center of each apple half.

Mix cornstarch and sugar and add boiling water to dissolve.
Cook until thickened and clear, stirring constantly.
Add drops of red food coloring and vanilla.
Pour or spoon sauce over apples and walnuts.

Sprinkle nutmeg over apples.
Bake at 400 degrees for about forty-five minutes or until apples are soft.
Dot the apples with marshmallows for the last minute of baking.

Delicious served warm or cold. (If served cold, Mother topped them with whipped cream instead of marshmallows.)

Serves six.

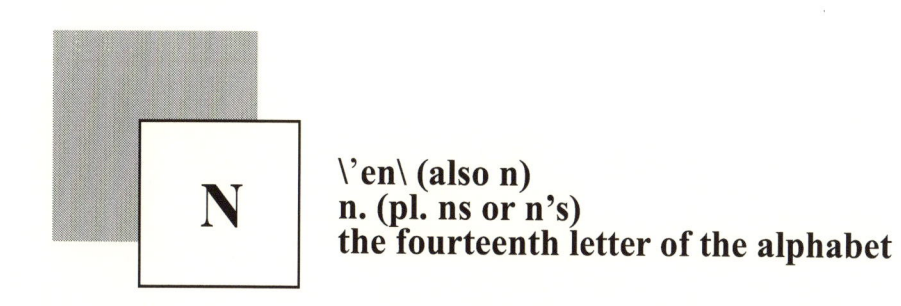

N \'en\ (also n)
n. (pl. ns or n's)
the fourteenth letter of the alphabet

NEIGHBORHOOD WITH A VIEW

Recipe: Peach and Berry Crisp

NEIGHBORHOOD WITH A VIEW

Dogwood (called Agony by runners), Parkway, Upland, and Alpine take you to the top of the steep hill north of Eastern Mennonite University (EMU). The street at the top, aptly named Hillcrest, runs north and south for about five blocks, bounded at each end by a cul-de-sac. Thirty-three houses line Hillcrest Drive, twenty on the western side of the street and thirteen on the eastern slope just below the crest.

From a realtor's perspective, the primary asset of a residence at this location is not the house itself but the outside expanse of land that can be seen toward Massanutten Mountain and the distant Blue Ridge on the east and the Allegheny Mountains on the west. Every home has "a room with a view." A friend once told me with a little envy that the car in our garage has a better view than many people. The first owner of our house ran a barber shop on the ground floor. His joke was to say to each patron who got out of the chair and stood by the window to put on his coat, "The haircut is free, but it'll cost you five dollars for the view!"

The landscape to the east still includes some farmland, but its foreground is dominated by the buildings of a retirement community, EMU's athletic fields, and the sparkling lake of evening lights we know as Harrisonburg. The western view of rolling hills and woodland patches is dotted with farm buildings and roaming cattle. Overhead, the sky-dome softly says that morning is coming by a glow of pinkness just above the Massanutten, and later, that day is done by the fanfare of red and gold behind the Alleghenies.

Most of the houses on Hillcrest are brick; the earliest was built in the 1940s, the more recent in the 1990s. Lawns are clean with well-clipped shrubbery and abundant flower beds. Trees give some shade but are planted in spots calculated not to obstruct the view. The owners live on their property, but many houses also have an apartment rented to young professionals or graduate students.

A few homes have high school or college age children, but most owners are age fifty or above. They are predominately white, middle-class people with professions such as doctor, pastor, business owner, professor, lawyer, journalist, social worker, nurse, real estate agent, and university administrator.

Of the thirty-three owners, Jay and I know the names of all but eight. Twenty homes are owned by people somewhat connected to a Mennonite congregation, ten by people now or once employed at EMU and thirteen by retired people.

The street is quiet and well-lit at night by street lamps. We keep our doors locked, but the neighbor across the street leaves her house open and goes away for the weekend. The most frequent visitors to Hillcrest are joggers, dog walkers, and lovers.

Our most imposing neighbor is the sixty-acre campus of EMU and its fifteen hundred students. Some occasionally take a short cut across our lawns, scream with residence hall pranks at night, and send their thunderous cheers up from the playing fields. Then they more than compensate by inviting us over for music and theatrical performances, lectures, athletic events, and almost-free meals in their cafeteria. We walk on their indoor and outdoor tracks and view the heavens east and west from their parklike campus hilltop. Perhaps more important than any of these perks is the infiltration of wider world views that EMU's Center for Justice and Peacebuilding and cross-cultural programs release into our community.

E. M. Forster's 1908 novel, *A Room with a View,* contrasts the symbolic differences between the restrictive society of Edwardian England (rooms) with the place of light and freedom (views) that Lucy Honeychurch finds in her travels in Italy. Static characters in the novel are conservative and uncreative and remain so. Dynamic characters are open and forward-thinking and have world views that change dramatically as the plot unfolds.

Neighbors on Hillcrest Drive literally have "a room with a view," a thirty-mile dynamic landscape seen from the windows of our rooms that changes with the weather and every season of the year. Do we also have the vista, the extensive mental view that embraces new people and ideas, that welcomes new opportunities to learn? Each of us must answer that question for him or herself.

Neighbors on Hillcrest are busy people, dashing off in our cars to work and volunteer, to committee meetings, and to social events at church. But neighbors on Hillcrest are also friendly people. "We must get together," we say as we chat along the street or across our flower beds. And sometimes we do get together.

Last winter, it snowed from dawn one Friday morning throughout the day, all night, and all day Saturday until about four o'clock when a weak western sun struggled through the clouds to let us know that the storm was over. Nearly two feet of snow covered everything, weighting the Blue Atlas cedar's branches to the ground, a low canopy over our front walk.

Early Saturday morning, I heard a scraping noise and looked out to see neighbor Jim Lofton clearing a path to our front door. I opened the door and asked, "What did we do to deserve such kindness?" "Well, I didn't want Jay to do it" was his reply. He came back several times during the day for periodic clean ups.

Around noon, Bonnie Lofton telephoned to invite us and three other neighbors to a potluck supper at their house. About six o'clock, we neighbors picked our ways carefully through the icy pathways to the Loftons' comfortable living room where we warmed around their wood fire.

Bonnie called us to stand and introduce ourselves in a circle around the dining room table laden with food. The Lofton household numbered two since James and Cara were away in school. Becky Benton, from the Lofton apartment, introduced herself as a diving coach at James Madison University. The Michael and Peggy Shenk household were six, including the Kenyan family who live in their apartment—Isaiah, Mary, Leonard, and Zoë. The Hostetter family added six more, including Mother and Grandmother Mildred, son Vaughn, and newest neighbors, son Eric and Janet and two of their three children. Kate Kessler, a writing teacher at JMU and her friend Joe Greenberg, an engineer from Charlottesville, were there, plus Jay and I, for a grand total of nineteen.

After Bonnie led us in "a prayer for a snowy day," we enjoyed the food, amazed at the bountiful and beautiful meal we could assemble even when snowbound and unable to make a trip to the grocery store. The vegetarians in the group found Bonnie's good bean soup, Kate's fresh fruit platter, and Janet's salad so satisfying. The meat lovers enjoyed Janet's barbeque sandwiches. The Kenyan family shared foods seasoned with the flavors of their homeland—a rice and beef dish and chai tea. Peggy Shenk's wonderful apple pie, and my peach and berry crisp provided ample dessert.

After the meal, we coaxed the Kenyan family into singing for us. They sang four or five vibrant songs in Swahili along with movement and clapping. The exuberant music of their homeland is one thing they miss very much, they told us. Another thing they miss is the respect shown to older people. The oldest person in the village is the "boss," the person with wisdom. We took a quick poll of our group and decided that Mildred should be the "boss." Truly she is a wise woman and genteel in every way, gracious characteristics that entitle her to be "neighborhood leader."

As we bundled up for the snowy walk home, we felt gratitude in our hearts for a warm fire, nutritious food, cultural diversity, and neighbors who are friends. Just before we left, Leo, the Loftons' happy-to-be-alive Labradoodle, bounded into the room to say goodbye!

Peach and Berry Crisp is one of my favorite desserts for a cold, snowy evening—or anytime! It carries well to potlucks or is a nutritious conclusion for a lighter meal served at home. Enjoy with ice cream!

PEACH AND BERRY CRISP

3 cups canned, sliced peaches, drained
3 cups frozen berries (any combination of blueberries, raspberries, or marionberries)

¼ cup of sugar
2 tablespoons cornstarch
½ cup water

3 tablespoons butter, melted
3 tablespoons canola oil
1 cup brown sugar
½ cup all-purpose flour
½ cup whole wheat flour
1 cup rolled oats
1 teaspoon cinnamon
½ cup walnuts, chopped (optional)

Arrange peaches in bottom of a seven-by-eleven-inch baking dish.

Mix sugar, cornstarch, and water in saucepan and cook until thickened and clear.

Add frozen berries to thickening and toss to cover. Spread evenly over peaches.

Mix oils, sugar, flours, oats, and cinnamon until crumbly. Add nuts and sprinkle topping over the fruit.

Bake in preheated oven at 375 degrees, thirty-five to forty-five minutes until top is golden and fruit bubbles.

Serves six to eight.

O \ˈō\ (also o)
n. (pl. os or o's)
the fifteenth letter of the alphabet

ORNAMENTAL TOUR

Recipe: Blueberry Oatmeal Muffins

Recipe: Orange-Blueberry Freezer Jam

OUCH AND OUNCE

My Granola

ORNAMENTAL TOUR

I have toured manor houses in England, such as Castle Howard and Blenheim Palace, where the guide uses white gloves if he touches anything. These tours usually end in the gift shop where sales add to the previously paid admission fee in order to maintain the estate.

This "tour" will not be as long or as gilded, nor will it cost anything. We will end in the dining room instead of the gift shop. However, there is this caveat. A thousand words are not as good as one picture. The reader's visual image of what I describe in a few words will be different than the art work itself—but imagination is often the beginning of new artistic expressions.

Our home, built in the late 1960s, was designed by the nephew-architect of the home economics professor who built it. The floor plan is functional and lends itself best to traditional style furnishings. Most of the walls are painted ivory, and the floors are covered with neutral honey-toned carpet. Sometimes we buy a new piece of furniture, always trying to select pieces that are consistent in size and color with earlier choices. I have been tempted to call a decorator—but never have—deciding instead to keep our décor simple and personal, our own expression of our fifty years of housekeeping.

So what is it after all that makes a home different than a furniture store? Without a doubt, it is the ornaments and accessories—the framed artwork, china and glassware, collections of books, pottery, plants, and curios—that personalize the space and remind one of the artist-creator, the giver, or the place of purchase.

This "tour of the ornaments" begins in our breakfast nook area. The original color woodcut hanging there, *Iris and Poppies,* is signed and numbered by the artist. Mervin Jules (1912-1994) was a realist born in Baltimore whose work often dealt with social themes; he was especially prolific as a printmaker. Jules exhibited in the United States and abroad, and his works are included in many public collections, including the Metropolitan Museum of Art.

We bought *Iris and Poppies* from a traveling art dealer in the 1980s. Six vibrant red poppies in the foreground backed by three bluish purple irises seem to be caught in motion from a stirring breeze. The strong blue and red colors of this favorite print have influenced our color choices time after time in the years since, as we have made selections of other artwork or furnishings for our home.

Ten small hen-on-the-nest collectibles in Depression glass colors of blue, red, amber, and green parade across the kitchen window ledge, leading the eye to a pair of roosters on the counter top. These flamboyant fellows are safely caged in a handmade platter and bowl set of Peggy Karr Glass, their brilliant colors fused between layers of clear glass. They are a gift from Ann. According to Italian legend, having a rooster in the kitchen is a symbol of luck, health, and prosperity—hopefully two roosters will add much warmth and happiness to the place!

One Christmas, Jim and Betty gave us *Butterflies and Foliage,* a scaled-down reproduction of a stained glass window created in 1889 by John La Farge (1835-1910). La Farge discovered opalescent glass and developed the technique of fusing bits of this glass without using leading. The shimmering beauty of *Butterflies and Foliage* against its background of blues is brought to life by the light on our sun porch at different hours of the morning.

The afternoon sun plays through another stained glass piece, this one original and custom-made by Carl and Jody Wright in their turn-of-the-century smokehouse studio in Martinsburg, West Virginia. We commissioned the twenty-by-sixty-two inch window in the 1990s to cover the glass panel in the foyer beside our front door. Using a traditional quilt block motif, they hand-cut the squares and triangles from textured West Virginia glass in patches of cobalt blue, deep red rose, turquoise, and white, and built an oak frame to hold it. We rented a van big enough to stand the piece on its side so it wouldn't break on its eighty-mile journey to our home.

A fourteen-inch tall bust of William Shakespeare, which I gave to Jay for his classroom many years ago, sits atop a bookcase in the office, looking down at the computer keyboard. "How many more plays could I have written if I had had one of those?" he wonders. This room is also the repository of our most precious piece of photography. Two-year-old twin daughters, Ann and Jill, smile for the Gitchell Studio photographer's toy in a nicely framed sixteen-by-twenty-inch oil-colored print. They are wearing identical soft pinwale teal-colored dresses with white lace collars made by their Grandma Heatwole. Their chubby little legs are cute in white knee socks and black patent leather shoes.

Two pieces of needlework have found places on our walls. A near-perfect cross-stitch sampler hangs in our bedroom, made for us as a twenty-fifth wedding anniversary gift by our dear friend, Irene Mullenex. When Uncle Elmer and Aunt Kazie Good from Seattle visited us in 1996, Aunt Kazie gave us one of her delicate pieces of lace tatting that I had framed against a blue velvet background and have hung in the hallway.

A gorgeous bowl of raku pottery made by Richard Reuter rests on a shelf in our bedroom. After the ceramic was fired in the kiln to over 2200 degrees, it was placed to cool in a chamber with Long Island sea grass soaked in sea water until its surface produced a shimmering rainbow effect. The turquoise, gold, and red-violet colors are perfectly matched in Barbara Gautcher's framed pastel drawing of a local landscape that hangs nearby.

Why do I love pottery? Maybe it meets the same inner need that inspired my great-great-grandfather Emanuel Suter (1833-1902) to build his pottery shop several years before the Civil War. Pottery is so elemental and so enduring. Even God himself used clay to shape the human form, his crowning work of creation.

A two-gallon crock made in Emanuel Suter's pottery sits in our living room. It was a birthday gift from Jay. It is unsigned, so we can't know for certain that his hands were on it, but I like to imagine them wet with slip as he cemented the handles in place before adding the blue leaves of decoration.

Another piece of pottery, this one on the coffee table, is the fourteen-inch platter made by Bill Campbell in his Cambridge Springs studio in Pennsylvania. It was given to me by my colleagues at MMA (now Everence) when I retired. The floral design divides the platter into quadrants; the petals are basically blue with highlights of red-violet bounded by a frosty light blue edge. Campbell specializes in functional work. "I merely try to cause a little celebration in everyday living," he writes, which is certainly what he does for me as I admire his spectacular colors and lustrous glaze.

Prayer Rug by Dennis Maust hangs on a panel beside the fireplace. It is a framed tessellation of 276 clay mosaic tiles that reflects the visual experiences Maust had while living overseas in Egypt and Pakistan. This mosaic is reminiscent of Persian rug patterns and has a central pattern that points heavenward like the tower of a minaret calling us to prayer. Design is created by the careful placement of the colored tiles in shades of light blue, mauve, stone, and black.

I don't buy on an impulse; if anything, I deliberate too long and then talk myself out of a purchase. The Delft porcelain wall hanging was lying on the dealer's table at the annual Harrisonburg Rotary antique sale. The attraction may have been the scrolled edges and floral flourishes on the oval shape or the blue and white cows walking downhill in perfect perspective or the ethereal blues of the Dutch countryside—or all of the above! I walked away, but I soon came back and paid far more than I ever imagined I would for love-at-first-sight. The panel is stamped, numbered, and signed by W. Reelofs. The pottery's mark dates it from about 1890, but beyond that, little is known. The dealer told us he bought it from the estate of Bob Walls, a curator of the Scottsville Museum in Albemarle County, Virginia.

Barbara Fast, professor in the Visual Arts Department of EMU, is a master of handmade paper pieces. One of her amazing early works has hung in our house for more than twenty-five years. Gusts of wind push the billowing cumulus clouds to the top of the impression. The suggestion of barren brown trees in the foothills of the distant blue mountains tells us that the season is winter; the pink hazes that tinge the horizon say that it is dawn and the sun will soon rise.

As we (my reader and I) have walked through this house, we have noticed various small pieces also, ornaments such as Ryan Mellinger's blown glass balls, Elizabeth Horst's Ukrainian egg, Grace Songolo's ceramic shell paperweight, and Dorothy Herrera's Native American story telling doll. These and others nurture the aesthetic in my spirit. I know I am privileged to live in the presence of this creativity.

Now it is time to take another beauty—the Wedgwood teapot Jay and I bought in Windsor—from its shelf and make our tea. We will sit at my new dining room table while we again enjoy my favorite color—blue—with good blueberry oatmeal muffins. We will "accessorize" them with orange-blueberry freezer jam, one bowl of ripe red strawberries and another of sweet whipped cream.

BLUEBERRY OATMEAL MUFFINS

1 and ⅔ cups quick-cooking oats
⅔ cup all-purpose flour
½ cup whole wheat flour
¾ cup packed light brown sugar
2 teaspoons ground cinnamon
1 teaspoon baking powder
1 teaspoon baking soda
¼ teaspoon salt

1 and ½ cups low-fat buttermilk
¼ cup canola oil
2 teaspoons grated lemon rind
2 large eggs

2 cups frozen blueberries
2 tablespoons all-purpose flour
Cooking spray

Preheat oven to 400 degrees.

Place oats in food processor; pulse five or six times or until oats resemble coarse meal. Place in a large bowl.

Spoon flours into dry measuring cups; level with a knife. Add flours and next five ingredients (through salt) to oats; stir well. Make a well in the center of the mixture.

Combine buttermilk and next three ingredients (through eggs). Add to flour mixture; stir just until moist.

Toss berries with two tablespoons flour and gently fold into batter. (This will keep them from turning the batter purple while they bake.)

Spoon batter into sixteen muffin cups coated with cooking spray; sprinkle cinnamon topping evenly over batter. (three tablespoons sugar, three teaspoons flour, one teaspoon cinnamon, one and a half teaspoon melted butter)

Bake at 400 degrees about sixteen minutes or until center springs back when lightly touched. Remove from pans immediately and place on wire rack.

ORANGE-BLUEBERRY FREEZER JAM

2 and ½ cups of sugar
1 medium navel orange
1 and ½ cups fresh blueberries
1 pouch (3 ounces) liquid fruit pectin

Place sugar in a shallow baking dish. Bake at 250 degrees for fifteen minutes. Meanwhile, grate one tablespoon peel from the orange. Peel, segment, and chop orange.

In a large bowl, combine the peel, chopped orange, mashed blueberries, and sugar; let stand for ten minutes, stirring occasionally.

Stir in pectin. Stir constantly for three minutes.

Ladle into clean jars or freezer containers. Let stand for twenty-four hours at room temperature. Refrigerate for up to three weeks or freeze.

Yield: four cups

OUCH AND OUNCE

"You look like your mother," people tell me sometimes. I agree because I have caught my unsuspecting self in a mirror and seen her expression, her fleshy cheek, and her smooth skin reflected back to me. But I silently disagree too because I know I have the hair texture, eye color, and crooked lower teeth of my father. Who I am physically is the mysterious mix of all those genes included in that one egg and sperm that was my conception along with the imprint of my environment in the years since.

My parents gifted me with a generally healthy childhood. The measles and an occasional cold or flu were all that prevented perfect attendance at school. When I was a high school sophomore, I survived a tiresome, but not serious, bout with infectious mononucleosis that kept me home in bed with an afternoon fever, swollen lymph nodes, and aching back muscles for about two weeks. The only prescription medicines I remember from those early years were some pills for a bladder infection and a salve to clear a ringworm lesion on my leg. Once a dentist put me to sleep with a gas "balloon" and pulled several stubborn molars for which I was rewarded a Betsy-Wetsy doll with a little tube that ran from her mouth to her diaper. I never broke a bone or had a hospital admission as a child.

My body withstood a healthy full-term pregnancy with twins and the busy years of family care and demanding career. Then as time moved on, I began to wonder what had happened to the strength that once enabled me to do so much. Dr. Andrew Weil, my health guru, writes, "Sixty is about the time that organs of the body begin gradually to fail, when the first hints of age-related disease begin to appear." (*Healthy Aging,* Alfred A. Knopf, New York, 2005, p. 3)

Ouch!

My first organ to fail was my uterus. In my midfifties, following a dilation and curettage (D&C) procedure, Dr. Witmer said, "You are healthy, but your uterus isn't." He found hyperplasia with atypical cells in the endometrium, and his solution was a hysterectomy and removal of my ovaries. I debated about the ovaries, but a friend had recently died of ovarian cancer, and I concluded that removal would mean one less kind of cancer to worry about.

January 1996 found me on the operating table. I had taken a pile of books to read during my five-day hospital stay. "You'll need six weeks' recovery time," I was advised. "Not me," I thought, "how could it take that long to recover my strength?" Truth be told, I did not read any of my books in the hospital, and I was glad for the six weeks' leave from my work.

Just as Dr. Weil predicted, other age-related disease developed in the next few years. My blood pressure numbers kept creeping up as did my triglycerides. "I'll take care of it with diet and exercise," I planned, but it didn't work. My father died at age eighty of an apparent heart attack, and his brother and several nephews had been stricken even earlier in their lives. It seemed wise to take Dr. Morgan's advice and begin a diuretic for my blood pressure and a statin for my cholesterol. Both have been effective.

In August 2000, we were vacationing in the Mariposa Valley, California, when I first became aware of a strange, burning sensation in my feet. The daytime temperatures were often more than one hundred degrees, so I paid little attention to the discomfort. Several months later, as the sensation persisted and I also experienced some tingling and numbness, I talked to my doctor and first heard the words "peripheral neuropathy."

Peripheral neuropathy is a disorder that involves the functioning of the nerves outside of the brain and spinal cord. They say it affects millions of Americans, mostly older adults. There are a variety of causes—the most common of which is diabetes. Other causes include alcoholism, vitamin deficiencies, certain medications, underactive thyroid, and inherited abnormalities. I was checked for diabetes, vitamin B12 deficiency, and thyroid activity. When all these tests came back negative, I was said to have idiopathic (of unknown cause) peripheral neuropathy.

My neurologist, Dr. Deputy, used a nerve conductor velocity test as a way of determining which nerves were causing the problem. He reported that the motor nerves seemed okay, making large motor activity such as walking possible. The inner, smaller sensory nerves were causing the painful sensations. He prescribed Neurontin, a drug with minimum side effects, to relieve my chronic nerve pain. Is it effective? How much better or worse would I be without it? So far, I have found the best medicine is keeping active. If I can divert my mind to other more interesting things, I can better ignore the pain. You can't focus on two things at the same time!

At age seventy, my ophthalmologist, Dr. Yoder, determined that the cataracts on both eyes had matured and were ready for surgery. His skillful hands replaced the lens on my right eye in March 2009. Inside the operating room, they gave me oxygen, placed a shield over most of my face, and washed the eye area. A bright light shone into my dilated eye, and I was instructed to look into the light, a hard assignment even though the eye was propped open. When the old lens was removed, the light swiveled and danced with red and blue colors, psychedelic and other worldly. Shortly, Dr. Yoder said he was finished, and the implant had gone "perfectly."

Back in the Ambulatory Surgery Center, I was given a cup of ginger ale, two Advil tablets, and instructions about my eye drops. For the rest of the day, I saw a snowy blizzard, but when the "storm" cleared, I saw colors brighter and clearer than I had seen for several years. I recalled stories of my grandfather lying in the hospital for days after his cataract surgery, his head between sand blocks. A month later, Dr. Yoder replaced the lens on my left eye.

Another eye incident occurred in February 2011 after I saw an unusual amount of smoky "floaters" in my right eye. A Harrisonburg ophthalmologist referred me to a retina specialist in Winchester. Dr. Carter confirmed that an unusual amount of vitreous gel had broken away and pulled a small tear in my retina. "Come with me," he said, and we walked down the hall to another small room where he zapped my eye twenty to thirty times with a laser light to hold the tear in place and prevent further detachment.

My "book doctor," Dr. Weil, warned me that things like this would happen after age sixty. And he did not promise that life would be easier in the decades ahead. I can expect the pain in my hip to continue or grow worse, more wrinkles to appear, more names to escape my memory, more reasons to visit the doctor and pharmacy. But his wise conclusion for the future is this:

> The best we can do—and it is a lot—is to accept this inevitability and try to adapt to it, to be in the best health we can at any age. . . . To age gracefully means to let nature take its course while doing everything in our power to delay the onset of age-related disease or in other words, to live as long and as well as possible, then have a rapid decline at the end of life. (Weil, p. 5)

"Doing everything in our power to delay the onset of age-related disease" brings me to the part *prevention* plays in my daily health journey.

Ounce!

Benjamin Franklin once said that "an ounce of prevention is worth a pound of cure." Too bad they don't bottle prevention and sell it at the drugstore; everyone must work out the formula and dosage for him or herself.

Another health resource book that has saved me many unnecessary trips to the doctor is *Taking Care of Yourself* by Donald M. Vickery, M. D. and James F. Fries, M. D., Perseus Books, 2001. The seven keys to health they outline are exercise, diet and nutrition, not smoking, alcohol moderation, weight control, avoiding injury, and professional prevention.

So let me examine my "ounce of prevention" on these seven keys. I would get high scores for not smoking and rarely using alcohol. I would get my lowest mark on exercise, to my shame. Walking has long been my exercise of choice, and in between lapses, I have done rather well, especially before neuropathy gave me another excuse. I have access to indoor and outdoor tracks in easy walking distance. Park Woods and the EMU campus offer other enjoyable, safe places to walk, and the hill of Dogwood Drive can quite quickly become aerobic. Ann has given me a pedometer, and I have good shoes. It is inexcusable that I find so many excuses. Sermon to myself concluded.

I have fought an often losing battle with the same twenty pounds for much of my adult life. Periodically, I choose a weapon—calorie counting, portion control, nothing white (flour, sugar, starch), occasional Scarsdale, or South Beach diets—and bring my weight under control. Might there be a connection between my not-so-diligent exercise and my desirable weight, I dare to wonder!

I almost always buckle my seatbelt and drive within the speed limits. We use smoke alarms in our house, have grab bars in the shower, keep floors clear of clutter, hold the stair rail as we go down. Avoiding injury is partly an exercise of common sense and caution, but there are unavoidable risks as well.

Professional prevention means working alongside the doctor for checkups with complete blood work and tests such as mammograms, colonoscopy, and bone density scan. I get an annual flu shot and have had the pneumonia and shingles vaccines. I take several over-the-counter supplements including fish oil, vitamin D3, and adult low dose aspirin.

When Dr. Zirkle examined the incision following my cesarean section way back in 1963, he complimented me on how well I was healing. "You can tell you've had good nutrition," he said. I was fortunate to have good farm-fresh food as I was growing up, and a healthful diet is still the ounce of prevention I emphasize most.

We fill our Farmers' Market bags with fresh fruit and vegetables, whole grain breads, and free-range eggs. Our grocery cart's load includes good oils like canola and olive, skim milk, and other low-fat dairy products. We read the labels and select the items with lowest sodium content, rejecting some entirely. At Costco, we buy fresh chicken and fish and a little red meat, all of which I repackage into small servings at home and freeze for later use. I usually bake my own desserts so that I can adjust the sugar, salt, and kind of flour and add no preservatives.

I believe another good "ounce" is to eat breakfast every morning. I look forward to my small bowl of homemade granola. In fact, if by some unexpected circumstance I should live to be one hundred, and they ask me the secret of my longevity, I will tell them that the credit goes to my granola!

MY GRANOLA

6 cups rolled oats
½ cup sunflower seeds

½ cup sliced almonds
½ cup chopped walnuts
½ cup sugarless coconut (optional)
½ cup wheat germ
½ cup dry milk powder
2 teaspoons cinnamon
1 teaspoon ginger

½ cup canola oil
½ cup honey
2 teaspoons vanilla

1 cup dried cranberries, raisins, or chopped apricots

Preheat oven to 350 degrees.

Place rolled oats in large, shallow baking pan, ten-by-sixteen-inches.

Toast oats for fifteen minutes.

Remove oats from oven and add all dry ingredients, sunflower seeds through ginger. Stir well.

Heat oil and honey in saucepan to boiling point. Remove from heat and stir in vanilla. Pour over dry ingredients and mix thoroughly.

Bake for fifteen to twenty minutes, stirring every three to five minutes until golden.

Do not over bake.

Cool in pan undisturbed.

Add cranberries or other fruit.

Freeze or store in airtight container.

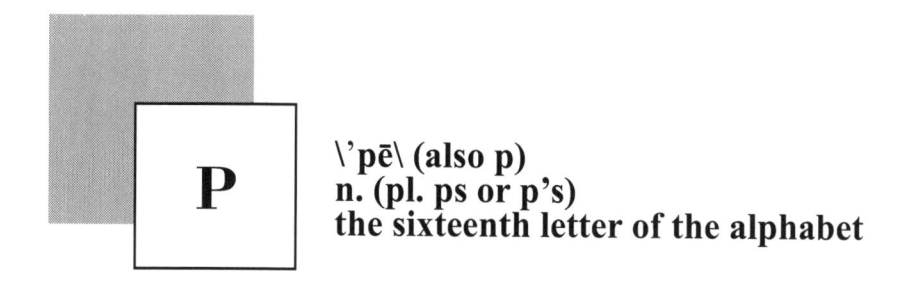

P \'pē\ (also p)
n. (pl. ps or p's)
the sixteenth letter of the alphabet

PARK VIEW MENNONITE CHURCH

Recipe: Hot Cross Buns with Cream Cheese Frosting

PHOTOGRAPHS

Recipe: Curried Chicken Divan

PARK VIEW MENNONITE CHURCH

"What is this place where we are meeting?" *

Three hundred voices singing in four-part a cappella harmony blend and lift the question to the skylights overhead. A sign outside answers their question, at least in part. It says this meeting place is Park View Mennonite Church. Mennonite? What is a Mennonite church?

I have attended a Mennonite church most of my life. My four grandparents were all Mennonite, but none of my many aunts, uncles, and cousins remained an adult member of the Mennonite church. My brother is no longer a Mennonite. Sometimes I ask myself why I alone carry this stream of my family's religious heritage forward. Have I chosen it, or did it choose me? Is my solitary stand significant for any reason? Is it an honor or a responsibility—or some rigid, tradition-bound inclination? Some "light" or some "blindness"?

I was baptized at age twelve by my own choice and with sufficient understanding of what that solemn rite signified. In the years since I have never seriously questioned my firm commitment to the way of Jesus, but as a young adult, I was less committed to the way of Menno.

When I was a junior in college, I took a class called Mennonite History and Thought taught by Professor Irvin B. Horst, a brilliant scholar who later held the chair of church history at the University of Amsterdam. In his class, I finally learned about my spiritual forefathers and foremothers, the "radical" Swiss and German Anabaptists (rebaptizers) of the sixteenth century. Menno Simons, a former Catholic priest and an early leader, gave his name to one group which believed firmly in the separation of church and state and committed themselves to follow Jesus each day as closely as possible to the way he outlined in the Sermon on the Mount (Matthew 5, 6, 7). This way required them to love their enemies, even the enemies of the state. Individuals joined this group of believers upon adult confession of faith and were rebaptized as an initiation to their new life of discipleship.

Today, the Mennonite Church numbers almost one and a half million members in seventy-five countries of the world, almost two-thirds of whom are outside North America. The vision statement of this church is that "God calls us to be followers of Jesus and by the power of the Holy Spirit to grow as communities of grace, joy, and peace so that God's healing and hope flow through us to the world."

Becoming and remaining a member of the Mennonite denomination was a pivotal decision that had a profound impact on the whole of my life. If I had chosen otherwise, it is unlikely that I would have married Jay, would live where I live, would have been employed where I worked much of my life, would have lived by the same set of values that influence my daily choices and actions.

*"What is this place where we are meeting?
Only a house, the earth its floor,
Walls and a roof sheltering people,
Windows for light, an open door."*

As the three hundred voices continue the hymn, my mind wanders back to the first time our family attended this particular congregation called Park View. It was a snowy Sunday in 1970 when the four of us slipped into a red-cushioned pew as visitors. The brick church building with white trim and steeple was about two years old at the time, and the clear glass windows on the north side looked out across open fields. I remember the comfortable, at-home feeling that pervaded as we worshipped that Sunday. Soon, we were regular attenders.

Over the next twenty years as the church grew in program and attendance, additional facilities were needed. A large addition was added on the north side, and the old sanctuary became the much needed larger fellowship hall. The new-again church building was dedicated in 1995.

*"We in this place remember and speak again what we have heard:
God's free redeeming word."*

The worship leader lights the peace lamp and calls us to worship, often with an antiphonal reading from scripture. Mennonites put great emphasis on reading and knowing the Bible, and there are readings from both the Old and New Testaments in most services. Since we view ourselves as a community of believers, there is wide participation from nonclergy. Children, youth, and adults are encouraged to lead in worship, and each person's gifts are valued.

Park View generally follows the liturgical calendar, and we recognize ourselves as part of the church universal when we consider the same scriptures as our evangelical sisters and brothers across the world. These scriptures usually suggest the theme for the morning service which is emphasized in the music and sermon.

Our family has known each of Park View's pastors as good preachers, as spiritual leaders, and as friends: Ira E. Miller (1953-1966), Harold G. Eshleman (1967-1974), A. Don Augsburger (1974-1980), Owen Burkholder (1981--1996), and Phil Kniss (1996 to the present). Without much struggle over the issue of women in ministry, the church accepted Shirlee K. Yoder as minister of Pastoral and Mutual Care in 1985 and Shirley Yoder Brubaker as associate pastor in 1991. In 2001, Barbara Moyer Lehman began service as associate pastor for Nurture and Pastoral Care; and in 2002, Ross Erb became associate pastor for children, youth, and families.

Following the sermon and offering, the church joins in prayer for the needs of members of the congregation as well as those beyond in our community and wider world. We remember our members who are away in service and each person by name who is having a birthday in the coming week.

A hymn follows the benediction. The blue hymnals go back into the racks along with the green ones and the purple ones. Mennonites love to sing, and they sing a lot. Unfortunately, joining the church does not bestow musical talent on a new member. I love the words of faith, but I sing softly and count on Jay's strong tenor to cover my worst notes. Four-part singing has been a long-standing tradition in the Mennonite Church. Once almost entirely a cappella, many churches today use organ, piano, and a variety of instruments. At Park View, many members have professional training. Our hymns reflect the sacred music of the wider world and are presented in various choral and instrumental ensembles.

The bread and wine of communion is served four or more times each year, a time of reflection and thanksgiving as we share the sacred symbols of Christ's body and blood, broken and spilt for all people.

"And we accept bread at his table, broken and shared, a living sign.
Here in this world, dying and living, we are each other's bread and wine.
This is the place where we can receive what we need to increase:
God's justice and God's peace."

Words from verse three of the hymn linger as we leave the sanctuary and head for the fellowship hall. "We are each other's bread and wine." Here, we have a cup of coffee or a cold drink as we greet visitors, admire a new baby, check on someone who has been ill, exchange news, plan for a meeting. Jay and I have made and served the coffee about once a month for many years. In the summertime, Jay's bouquet of roses on the serving counter gives a greater lift than the caffeine!

When the buzzer sounds, we join our Colloquy classmates downstairs for an hour of study and sharing. This class began about 1980 when we and two other couples were asked to start a group committed to friendship and fellowship. About ten of the original twenty members remain, but the total has grown to over fifty. This is my "church within a church," the unit where we truly are "each other's bread and wine." We joy and sorrow with each other through life's circumstances; we know when members are absent; we question and challenge each other; we learn and grow together; and we have fun. Monthly social activities have included trips to Washington DC, coffeehouse talent events, hikes in Shenandoah National Park, curry suppers, service projects, Christmas parties, and more potluck meals than we can count!

"This is the place where we can receive what we need to increase: God's justice and God's peace."

As chair of the Missions Commission, a post I have held from 2004 to the present, I have the opportunity of sharing in the church's efforts to promote "God's justice and God's peace" beyond the walls of our own building. The commission of nine members works together to coordinate various local and church-wide service programs and to prepare the annual missions spending plan for the PVMC budget, a current amount of one hundred thirty-two thousand dollars divided among thirty-plus agencies, not including generous above-budget giving.

In our world and in our neighborhood, many literally hunger and thirst and go without shelter. The work of the Missions Commission ministers to some of these needs. On the third Sunday of each month, Park View members carry in grocery bags full of nonperishable foods for the local Patchwork Pantry. In 2007, a team of six was sent from Park View to rural Kenya to assist local farmers in the construction of two concrete sand dams that conserve water under a deep layer of sand in a region that suffers several months of severe drought each year. This project was done in cooperation with MCC, the relief and service agency of the Mennonite Church. For several years, PVMC has opened its doors to provide meals and overnight shelter for up to forty homeless persons through HARTS (Harrisonburg and Rockingham Thermal Shelter), sharing in this ministry with other local churches. These are examples of numerous efforts we make to aid those in need. We believe that Jesus literally meant for his followers to give food and cold water in his name.

* "What is this place," *Hymnal: A Worship Book,* Mennonite Publishing House, Scottdale, Pennsylvania, 1992, p. 1.

As I write this description of my church, we are in the season of Lent, the forty-day journey of reflection and repentance prior to Easter and the celebration of new life and renewal. The rough boards of the cross at the front of Park View Mennonite Church are draped in purple. Plans are being made for the activities of Holy Week, including the Good Friday night Tenebrae service when the sanctuary is stripped of all decoration, and we sit in darkness, remembering.

Hot Cross Buns are typically eaten on Good Friday and during the season of Lent. Stories abound about the origin of the Hot Cross Bun. Some say it dates back to the twelfth century when an Anglican monk placed the sign of the cross on the buns he was baking to honor Good Friday. Supposedly, this pastry became the only thing permitted to enter the mouths of the faithful on this holy day.

I clipped this recipe from a newspaper article many years ago and share it here with a few adaptations. Working with yeast breads, a symbol of life and resurrection, is particularly meaningful during the Easter season.

HOT CROSS BUNS with Cream Cheese Frosting

2 cups all-purpose flour
2 packages active dry yeast
½ cup granulated sugar
1 teaspoon salt
1 and ½ teaspoons cinnamon
½ teaspoon nutmeg

1 cup milk
½ cup butter

3 eggs, lightly beaten
1 cup currants or raisins
⅓ cup candied orange peel (optional)
3 additional cups of flour (more, if needed)

1 egg yolk mixed with two tablespoons water

Combine two cups of flour, yeast, granulated sugar, salt, and spices in a large mixer bowl.

In a separate bowl, heat the milk and butter to very warm (120 to 130 degrees). Add to flour mixture. Beat on medium speed of electric mixer for one minute.

Add eggs. Beat another minute.

Stir in currants, orange peel, and enough remaining flour to make dough easy to handle.

Turn dough out onto lightly floured work surface and knead until smooth and elastic, about five minutes, adding additional flour as needed. Place in a buttered bowl, turning to butter the top. Cover; let rise in warm place until doubled in bulk, about one hour. Punch down dough and knead again for several minutes; turn onto lightly floured work surface.

Line a large baking pan (or pans) with parchment paper. Divide dough into twenty-four equal pieces (in half, half again, etc.,). Shape each portion into a ball and place on baking sheet, about an inch apart. Cover with a clean kitchen towel and let rise in a warm, draft-free place until doubled in size, about one and a half hours.

When the buns have risen, take a sharp or serrated knife and carefully slash each with a cross. Brush each bun with the egg yolk and water mixture.

Bake in preheated oven at 375 degrees, twenty to twenty-five minutes or until golden brown. Remove from pans. Cool on wire rack. When the buns are cool, pipe or paint frosting on each in the shape of a cross.

Cream Cheese Frosting

3 ounce package cream cheese, softened
1 cup confectioners' sugar
1 and ½ teaspoon lemon or orange zest
1 teaspoon milk

PHOTOGRAPHS

Miss Ella

Our three file boxes with hanging folders full of photographs contain no image of Miss Ella. I must rely on my childhood memory of her petite frame and very white hair neatly drawn back and pinned in a small knot, her prim mouth of pearly white teeth and her enveloping white apron stuck with several safety pins.

Miss Ella lived across the road from my Keezletown bungalow in a large frame house with vestiges of an earlier grandeur. Her family members included demented Aunt Sally who sat on the kitchen rocker munching sugar cookies, feeble-minded sister Nancy who had been violated and bore an illegitimate son in her youth, and bachelor brother, Mr. Paul, who drove away in his black suit and black coupe to work somewhere every day. Chippy, a wiry terrier with one blind eye, completed the unusual household.

Upstairs in an unused bedroom, I fantasized about the elegant evening gowns that hung in a closet. Miss Ella wore these when she attended meetings of her society, the Evening Star. In the parlor downstairs, leather-bound volumes filled the bookshelves beside the itchy horsehair sofa. Outside, the porch swing was good for a few arcs, and the hollyhock blossoms could be fashioned into dolls with pink skirts.

It was a place of intrigue and very inviting to a child with some imagination. Mother had no fears and allowed me to run over often to "see Miss Ella." I was there one evening when it was time for Miss Ella to make supper, and it was then that I had my first memorable cooking lesson. I was maybe six or seven.

Miss Ella decided to have potato soup. She let me wash a few potatoes she had dug earlier from her garden. She trusted me with the sharp paring knife as I peeled them and cut them into little cubes. When the kitchen range was hot, we watched them bubble in the little pan until they were soft, then added butter and milk contributed by Miss Ella's cow and some salt and pepper from the cupboard. I had a little sip of my creation before I ran home to tell Mother.

I could cook! I was empowered!

Mrs. Conrad

I often visited the homes of my friends, cousins, and neighbors—houses with interiors that looked similar to my own. But what about those homes belonging to Harrisonburg's business and professional residents, houses that were kept clean by "help" who lived in some other more lowly place?

What did the houses of wealthy people look like inside? The answer to that question, as well as the lure of a little extra spending money, led me to accept Mrs. Conrad's offer of employment—my first job!

Mrs. Conrad and her attorney husband, whom I rarely saw, lived in a large brand-new split-level house with wall-to-wall champagne beige shag carpet. A small putting green lay outside the sliding glass doors on the back lawn where Mrs. Conrad practiced a few strokes occasionally. A "garden boy" took care of the large lawn and the shrubbery.

Mrs. Conrad's efforts to appear younger than her actual age were only partially successful. The unnatural color of her thinning auburn hair was a shade dark for her translucent, fair skin and age spots mingled with the freckles on her arthritic hands and nails painted silver. Her clothing might be described as jaunty. On a particular day, she might wear black toreador pants, an olive-green blouse with a sailor collar, red belt, and red shoes. Yet her slim figure and erect posture were striking. She was bossy in a friendly sort of way. Her voice reminded me of applesauce—sweet and smooth but tangy.

The Saturday work had its routines, beginning with the upstairs bedrooms where I stripped the beds—he and she occupied separate rooms—and remade them with clean sheets. Then I dusted and ran the vacuum cleaner in all three bedrooms. Mrs. Conrad was using the guest bedroom to write her novel. The lunch menu was fairly predictable too. Mrs. Conrad often scrambled us each an egg that she served with toast, a piece of fruit, and a glass of milk. She carried her lunch into the dining room, and I ate mine at the kitchen table.

Mrs. Conrad also employed an African-American "girl" who usually came to work on Tuesday, but one Saturday, she was there too, and we pursued our separate tasks throughout the morning, our paths seldom crossing in the large house. It was in the early 1960s, and this was the South. I spent the morning teasing my mind with Mrs. Conrad's lunchtime dilemma. When it was time to serve the scrambled eggs, what would she do? She could serve us both in the kitchen because we were both hired help. On the other hand, she could serve Rose in the kitchen and take me into the dining room with her since we were both white. Or perhaps she would stagger our lunch breaks. When the eggs and toast were ready, she did the one thing I had not considered. She joined us, and we all three ate at the kitchen table! Assuming that I was the most religious of the group, she invited me to offer a prayer of thanks!

Around Christmas one year, I walked into the living room and saw two mink stoles casually flopped over an armchair. As I stood and admired their elegance, Mrs. Conrad entered the room and announced that she was undecided between the silver and the autumn haze one and wanted me to model each of them for her. They felt so good—a floating softness! Does the little mammal who wears this fur on an everyday basis enjoy the luxury, I wondered, or does it have to be plundered to be so appreciated?

One year when Jay gave me a piano for Christmas, Mrs. Conrad, who had once been a piano teacher, decided that I should stay a half hour longer after my work was finished for a free piano lesson. Each week, I sat with her at her blond piano while the bust of Robert E. Lee watched my uncertain fingers.

On June 10, 1961, the morning of my wedding day, Mrs. Conrad entertained me, my bridesmaids, my mother, and the mother of my maid of honor at a "Bride's Breakfast." The dining room table was set with flowers, lace placemats, and the good china. The main entree was an individually baked egg dish topped with steamed shrimp.

That occasion also marked the end of my four years as a domestic employee. My goals were basically achieved. I had earned enough spending money because Mrs. Conrad was generous and paid more than the going rate. The new modern house was a pleasing place to work, and my employer's lifestyle opened a window on a world different from my own.

Shirley

When I had room for elective classes in college, I selected design and crafts, art in everyday life, and art appreciation. I carried a sketchbook to Europe the summer of 1960 and attempted some charcoal sketches of the pigeons in Trafalgar Square as well as a few monuments that were more willing to stand still while I drew! As a young mother, I somehow found a little time to audit painting and composition and to enroll in continuing education classes in watercolor and drawing.

My most important drawing lessons began the fall of 2001 when my friend, Shirley Stoltzfus, invited me to lunch to celebrate my recent retirement. "What are you going to do with your time now?" she asked me.

I mentioned several possibilities, including an interest in learning how to draw better. Instantly, her eyes sparkled with enthusiasm, and she confessed that she shared the same goal. Before we had finished our iced tea that afternoon, a seven-year-long drawing course was born. We agreed to meet the following Wednesday morning at her home to show each other some of our earlier work and to make our plan.

Since Shirley and I had both been teachers, it wasn't hard to plan a curriculum. We knew we needed a textbook and settled on *The New Drawing on the Right Side of the Brain* by Betty Edwards (Jeremy P. Tarcher/Putnam, 1999). Edwards encouraged us by writing that any person who can print legibly has ample dexterity to draw well, but she warned us that drawing is not about the hands but the *eyes* and the *brain*, particularly the right brain that functions in nonverbal, spatial, and holistic ways. We faithfully assigned ourselves her exercises, met weekly for several hours to "show and tell," and were rewarded by seeing our skills continue to improve. When we finished the Edwards text, we chose another, and another through five books. Our fat portfolios prove our persistence!

As the weeks went by, Shirley and I spent more and more of our time chatting about news and concerns. Always when I brought my drawings to her kitchen table, she greeted me with warm smiles and a prevailing optimism. When she came to my house, I noticed how carefully she walked from her car to my front door. I learned that she had a congenital curvature of the spine, complicated now by stenosis, a narrowing of the open spaces within the spine that put pressure on the nerves in the spinal column. Standing for a time *hurt* and ultimately forced her to give up her volunteer work and many other activities she truly loved, including our drawing lessons. Still, her eyes sparkled, and she insisted on knowing about me and what I had been doing lately.

Drawing lessons took second place to other lessons Shirley was inadvertently teaching me. She became my best example of the scripture which says, "We rejoice in our sufferings, knowing that suffering produces endurance, and endurance produces character, and character produces hope . . ." (Romans 5: 3,4 RSV) Shirley's ability to rejoice, even in pain, came full circle to result in her spirit of hope and optimism.

So why, I ask myself, has my attraction to the art of drawing persisted for so many years? When I am absorbed in the *process* of drawing, I experience an altered state of consciousness, of being concentrated and "at one" with whatever I am drawing. I can dismiss the clock and other distractions. On finishing the drawing, I do not feel tired but energized and refreshed. It is a kind of meditation.

In 2004, I went with Jay to a writers' conference at Saint John's College in Santa Fe, New Mexico. One morning while Jay was in class, I took my Bible, my colored pencils, and my sketchbook and sat on the balcony overlooking the majestic vistas of the Sangre de Cristo Range. In response to that overwhelming beauty, I literally drew the words of Psalm 36:5, "Your love, O Lord, reaches to the heavens, your faithfulness to the skies" into my sketchbook and added a light background of the distant mountains and expanse of sky. This was a profound experience of worship made intensely more memorable by the aid of my pencils. I thank Shirley for helping to make that possible.

Liang

In 2011, the Chinese census recorded more than 1.3 billion people. What are the chances that one face would emerge from that crowd and become our friend? That face belonged to Mr. Liang Yong. When we answered the door bell on September 1, 2011, we were face-to-face with a tall, good-looking man about thirty-five years of age. He had traveled from Zigong, a city in the Sichuan Province, to spend six months at Eastern Mennonite University as part of the Visiting Scholar Program sponsored by Mennonite Partners in China. He was to live in our efficiency apartment during that time.

We invited him into our living room where he sat rather tentatively toward the front of his chair as we exchanged welcome greetings and bits of information about our families. Mr. Liang had left his wife and five-year-old son at home in Zigong where his wife was also a teacher. He had come to improve his English, although it was fairly good already. In a blog that he shared with us later, he wrote, "I was full of uneasiness, suspicions, and a little bit of excitement. I know it is a different of country of different culture with everybody here behaving and treating the fellows differently. I knew people here didn't care much about others . . . Peggy and Jay was the landlord of the house, which I mean the word mainly involves or reminds people of rules, discipline, rent, and conflicting status."

The next morning, Liang appeared at our door again, smiling and pleasant and apologizing that he had forgotten to give us his gift. He handed us two small cloth bags, one red and one green, closed at the top with a drawstring. Inside each were about twenty small, hard "cookies" wrapped in tissue paper with instructions written entirely in Chinese characters. It was our turn to be "full of uneasiness, suspicions, and a little bit of excitement!"

"It's tea," he told us. "Pu-erh tea." Later, our Internet search yielded a little more information. Pu-erh tea is a wonder tonic that originates from the Yunnan Province of China, cultivated from wild broad leaf tea trees. Traditionally, the tea was pressed raw into cakes and then vaulted for up to a hundred years to gain its fermentation status, but now, an artificial aging process requires only twenty to forty days. The older the tea, the more expensive it is, with some tea cakes selling for thousands of dollars. Pu-erh is coveted for its preventative and curative properties and has been used to reduce cholesterol, lower blood pressure, attack free radicals, improve eyesight, and inhibit "internal dampness." A taste for its distinctive flavor would need to be cultivated, we decided.

Several days later, we spent an afternoon orienting Liang to the city and community. We studied maps before taking a drive on some of the area highways. In downtown Harrisonburg, we got bus maps from the Visitor Center, visited the public library, and enjoyed a pot of oolong tea, sandwiches, and conversation at a little tea shop.

In late October, it snowed. Shortly, Liang was at the door looking exuberant! In south central China, where he lives, they see a little snow about once a decade. He had taken pictures and sent them to his family by Skype and heard his son say, "Dad! I want to be there!" In his blog, Liang gave us the credit: "They prayed for the snow because I seldom had snow in my hometown and suggested to pile a snow man, naming it Liang Luojia for my son."

During his stay, we ate together in restaurants several times, and I occasionally invited him to join us at our table with other guests. He showed us videos of his home and family. Sometimes he asked for help in expressing his thoughts in English for a paper he was writing. He remembered us at Christmas, and we remembered his Chinese New Year. Jokingly, he called us his "Mennonite parents."

As time for his departure came, we realized how fond we had become of him and invited him on one of his last mornings for American coffee (which he liked) and a coffee cake. About this occasion, he wrote, "We talked a lot, hoping that we would see each other in the future. Before the conversation was done, to my surprise, they took out gifts for me, my wife, and my son, respectively . . . I was deeply moved that they took me as a good friend whom they will probably not meet again. How important and serious they treated the friendship between us! Thank you, Mennonite heart."

Effie and Her Parents

Sometimes Friday evening calls for comfort food in a cozy diner. Marti may call and wonder if we can meet them for supper at Mrs. Thomas's in Dayton. On one of those occasions, we arrived first and waited at a table until the Eads family arrived. Soon, three-year-old Effie came bouncing back the aisle but suddenly stopped to ask her mother a question. "Is this 'public'?" she wondered. "Yes," Marti responded, "this is 'public.'" Then Marti explained to us that she had put a puff of face powder on her own nose before leaving the house, and Effie wondered why. "Because ladies do that sometimes before they go out in public," Marti had replied. The word puzzled Effie all the way to the restaurant and waited to be clarified.

From very early, Effie's verbal abilities have been phenomenal, and she learned to read before age four. When she doesn't understand a word, she asks. What does *dona nobis pacem* mean? Why do they call him "president," she queries.

When we visit for a meal, we often take Effie a small gift. Later, she dictates a thank you note which Marti transcribes verbatim. I have saved many of these because they are so delightful.

"Dear Aunt Peggy and Uncle Jay,

Thank you for the Play-Doh factory, and
you are so generous that I even talk your eyes off.

Your friend,
Effie"

Marti and Christopher moved to Harrisonburg in fall 2003 for Marti to become a professor in the language and literature department at EMU. She and Jay enjoyed their work as colleagues, while Christopher and I made ourselves useful as "spouses" in the background. About the ages of our own children, they soon became almost family to us. With Baptist, Catholic, and Episcopal backgrounds, they were curious about Mennonites, and Christopher once called Jay "the quintessential Mennonite." An architect with a flair for many things, including design and calligraphy, he surprised us with an original framed gift containing this blessing written by our founder, Menno Simons, 1554:

Herewith I commend you to God.
May he guide your feet upon the way of peace,
and lead you in the unadulterated pure knowledge of his eternal, saving truth.

Marti and Christopher are both good cooks, and we delight in their spontaneous invitations to supper. When we are all seated at the table, we hold hands and begin:

One:	The Lord be with you.
All:	And also with you.
Effie:	Let us pray!

On one of those evenings, Marti served curried chicken divan, a delicious one-dish meal.

CURRIED CHICKEN DIVAN

2 cooked chicken breasts, cut into quarters or smaller
2 ten-ounce packages broccoli spears
1 ten-ounce can cream of chicken soup
1 small can sliced mushrooms
½ cup mayonnaise
⅓ cup evaporated milk
⅓ cup shredded American cheese

1 teaspoon lemon juice
½ teaspoon curry powder

1 tablespoon melted butter
½ Ritz crackers, crumbled

Arrange cooked broccoli spears in a lightly greased two-quart casserole; top with chicken and mushrooms.

Combine soup, mayonnaise, milk, cheese, lemon juice, and curry powder. Stir well, and pour over chicken. Top with buttered crumbs.

Bake at 350 degrees for twenty-five to thirty minutes.

Serves five or six.

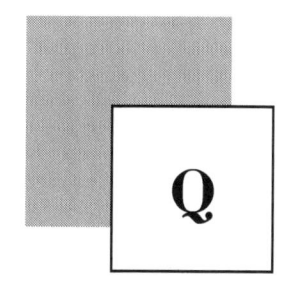

Q \'kyü\ (also q)
n. (pl. qs or q's)
the seventeenth letter of the alphabet

QUILT STORY

Recipe: Five-Cheese, Five-Vegetable Lasagna

QUILT STORY

The upstairs bedrooms of our old farmhouse were really cold on winter nights. My room had no heat except the little that escaped through the ceiling vent from the living room below. Never lingering long, I quickly sandwiched myself between the flannel sheets and shivered until my body heat and the bedcovers worked together to become a cozy nest. Somewhere above the flannel sheet and below the yellow chenille counterpane lay an old woolen comforter, pieced in four-inch blocks and knotted with yarn at each corner connecting point. The squares were probably cut from old coats, somber grays and greens and browns, not pretty but very practical. It kept me from freezing to death!

In my mother's cedar chest was another bed covering we never used no matter how cold the night. The pink and green Dahlia quilt was made by Mother and Grandma Suter during the Depression before Mother was married. The quilt has twenty pink twelve-inch dahlias, each with smaller white petals gathered into a pale green center. The dahlias are neatly appliquéd on a green background with a border of alternating pink, green, and white blocks. The main construction was done by machine, certainly a treadle with foot pedal. It is a thin all-cotton quilt, probably using a white cotton blanket as batting; these could be bought for as little as ninety cents in those days. Grandma Suter and Mother's tiny stitches, eight or ten to an inch, embellish the quilt in feather circles and diamond hatching. Of interest to me is that the quilt is not a patchwork quilt even though these were Depression days. The colors were chosen, and the fabric was purchased for this particular quilt. It was made as an artistic expression, not for utilitarian purposes. It is the only item I own that includes the work of my grandmother's hands.

The woolen comforter and the Dahlia quilt are remnants of American history, part of a much larger past that old bed coverings reveal. These quilts and comforters tell about the ups and downs of financial conditions, home construction that did not include central heating, and the preferences and fads of the time, often shown by the colors and patterns chosen. How I wish the Dahlia quilt could also tell me what it heard my mother and grandmother saying to each other as they worked together around the quilting frame!

Mother kept up her quilting skills by attending the monthly sewing circle of her church where she helped to make quilts for relief. As a thrifty homemaker, she saved fabric leftovers from our dresses and once pieced a string quilt, but she didn't enjoy the machine work nearly as much as the quilting. I often watched as she used the thimble on the middle finger of her right hand to push her number 10 betweens needle through all three layers in tiny running stitches. Nobody removed her stitches after she left the quilting party—she was a good quilter!

When Mother retired and had time, I seized my opportunity and commissioned her to make two whole cloth quilts for me. The three layers—a top made from a solid piece of creamy white fabric, a very thin Mountain Mist batting, and a backing—are all quilted together in a pattern that becomes the decoration. One of these two quilts is quilted with a grapevine medallion in the center and backed in blue fabric. The other is quilted with a pineapple medallion and backed in yellow fabric. Presently, they are part of my stash; but one day, they will become gifts for my daughters, Ann and Jill. We displayed these two quilts during the visitation hours before Mother's funeral where they rightfully received the acclaim that was their due.

My own quilt story did not begin until 1993 after I had retired from full-time work. Jay encouraged me to begin the quilt that I had long vowed I would someday make, while Mother was able to quilt it for me. Aunt Hazel, another outstanding quilt maker, suggested I begin with a Double Irish Chain. I bought *The Irish Chain Quilt* by Blanche Young and Helen Young Frost, and the book became my teacher, a basic instructor for this and future projects.

When I had planned my quilt, I made a trip to Clothes Line (now Patchwork Plus), a good fabric shop for quilters in Dayton, Virginia. There I purchased a rotary cutter, a large cutting mat, and a twenty-four-by-six-inch plastic grid and ruler with a handle. Jay took a fancy to these tools and offered to cut out my quilt. He has since become my precision cutter, accurate to the eighth of an inch!

My Double Irish Chain has a white background, two chains of cherry red, and one chain of navy with small red flowers. I pieced the quilt using the strip method and continuous stitching, then pinning every corner to be as accurate as possible. Mother quilted a tulip design in the open block and a chain of tulips in the border. I was so proud of my finished product that I displayed it on our bed for several years before I realized that the sun was fading the blue blocks.

But I was hooked! I found that every stage of the process was rewarding! First, there was the creative challenge of selecting the design and adapting it to my own personal tastes. Then came the trip to the store to choose fabrics with the right colors and patterns. Next, I delighted in the tactile experience of handling the good quality cottons as the blocks were stitched. The final reward was seeing the transformations that unfolded as the blocks were assembled into the completed top; the designs were lifted and enhanced by the quilting; and the edges were bound to complete the work.

After the Double Irish Chain was finished, I decided to take my work to the next level by enrolling in a sampler class taught by Mary Beery, an Old Order Mennonite lady recognized as an expert quilt maker. I made a number of the sampler blocks she demonstrated and turned them into sofa cushions rather than a quilt.

My next big project was to make two queen size tops which Mother quilted as Christmas gifts for Jill and Ann. When I selected the fabric for Jill's Log Cabin, it was Mary Beery's discerning eye that chose the exactly right red for the hearth-center block. Ann helped to select the fabrics for her Eight Point Star, a colorful portrayal of the Shenandoah Valley landscape with its purple mountains, rolling green fields, blue skies, little red barns, and of course, the stars.

In 1996, with a thirty-fifth wedding anniversary to celebrate, I decided to make a commemorative quilt. Aunt Hazel loaned me her old templates for the Double Wedding Ring, a pattern that first came into prominence during the Great Depression. My Double Wedding Ring contains seventy-two rings: thirty-six in reds and thirty-six in blues. I tell Jay that he is the red (active and outgoing), and I am the blue (quiet and reflective). The overlapping arcs are joined to a tea-toned background center and insert in which Mother quilted wild roses and small interlocking wedding rings. Now with a fiftieth wedding anniversary on the horizon, there may be another commemorative quilt in the pipeline. It's always a quilt maker's prerogative to dream about the next project!

With a growing stash of fabric scraps, the only thing to do was make scrap quilts! Making something out of "nothing" is more fun than anything! And so were created "Picket Fence," "Garden Maze," "Many Trips Around the World," "Stairway to Heaven," "Sister's Choice" and three throws, "Winter and Summer and Autumn Birds in Air." "Christmas Star" belongs in this category, although I bought the red and green batiks specifically for this quilt.

Sometimes a delightful surprise comes one's way! Jay and I were attending the quilt auction at the annual Virginia Mennonite Relief Sale. When Jay discovered how much I admired a little Crazy Quilt on display, he was determined to make it mine and kept nodding to the auctioneer until it was! We later met the quilter, Dorcas Steffen Hansbury, who was a home economics teacher somewhere in the Tidewater area. A dressmaker had given her scrap pieces of silks and velvets for her students' projects. Knowing that these fabrics would be too challenging for beginners, she used them herself to make Crazy Quilts for relief sales.

In the latter years of the nineteenth century in America, Crazy Quilts became very popular. The name of these quilts refers to the random, irregular pattern of needlework that is reminiscent of crazed china whose glaze is cracked in unpredictable patterns. These quilts were refined, luxury items of rich fabrics, usually finished with decorative embroidery. They were show pieces, often a small size, and used as a throw for the parlor couch. My little Crazy Quilt is made of satins and velvets in jewel-tone colors of pink, lavender, red, blue, and green. It has a dark green velvet backing and is embroidered in a variety of threads with feather, herringbone, blanket, and other stitches, little flowers, and French knots.

The Virginia Quilt Museum opened its doors in downtown Harrisonburg in August 1995. The museum is housed in the historic Warren-Sipe House, completed by Warren in 1855, a grand brick structure with large rooms, twelve-foot high ceilings, and a lovely center hall staircase. Sipe, a later owner, added mahogany fireplace frames and inlaid wooden floors. In addition to housing a permanent collection of several hundred quilts, the museum offers three major exhibits each year.

One Sunday afternoon, Jay and I stopped to see an exhibit and met friendly Paula Caldwell, a board member and the volunteer docent for the day. When she learned of my interest in quilts, she invited me to become a member and volunteer at the museum. I enjoy volunteering at the receptionist desk or in the museum shop about once a month.

One day, the first director, Joan Knight, told me she was looking for a variety of Log Cabin quilts for an upcoming exhibit. I told her about my Colorado Log Cabin, and she asked to see it. When I took it to her, I decided to also take my Pineapple Log Cabin for good measure. Imagine my delight when she informed me that the committee had decided to hang both quilts in the upcoming show, "Around the Hearth." The exhibit opened in May 2006 and showed for four months. Each of my quilts now proudly bears a label with the museum logo stating that it was exhibited at the Virginia Quilt Museum.

The Log Cabin is my favorite quilt pattern. Its basic piece is the small square at the center, the "hearth," that is often cut from red or yellow fabric to symbolize the warmth of home. Around the hearth, strips of lighter and darker shades build the log cabin. The quilt blocks can be assembled in many different layouts, creating limitless variety in the final presentation.

I pieced my Colorado Log Cabin in 1995 using light blues and deeper reds with a white eight-point star where each block connects to its neighbor. The large queen-size quilt is set in a diamond pattern and was quilted by my mother, Dorothy Heatwole.

The pattern for my Pineapple Log Cabin was based on an antique quilt made in 1920, possibly in Missouri. Because of the precise piecing needed, I used the foundation method, sewing each strip to a large paper square that I later peeled away. The colors are ivory and gold (like a pineapple!), and it was quilted in 2005 by Mother's friend, Minnie Carr.

My daughter, Jill, has become the most recent quilt maker in our family—Grandma Pearl, Mother Dorothy, Peggy, and now Daughter Jill. When her children were preschoolers and she had time for projects at home, she began, like I, with a Double Irish Chain of pink colors and flowers for Becky's bed. "A Summer Walk" and "Indian Blanket" were made for Nate and Tim, respectively, featuring birds and horses. For her own and Craig's bed, she used the Log Cabin pattern to create an impressionistic seasonal cycle, using her artistic bent to interpret the calendar in winter blues, spring pinks, summer yellows, and autumn deep reds. Light blues unify the quilt and suggest the heavens above us in all seasons.

Putting together a dish of lasagna is reminiscent of preparing a quilt for the frame! The three layers of pasta in this vegetable lasagna become the backing, batting, and top of the "quilt," and the colorful vegetables give it pattern and variety. This recipe makes twelve ample servings, and some could be frozen to pull out for a quick supper when a time-consuming quilting project is under way!

FIVE-CHEESE, FIVE-VEGETABLE LASAGNA

1 package (10 ounces) frozen chopped spinach, thawed and well-drained
⅓ cup of butter
½ cup all-purpose flour
3 cups milk
½ cup grated Parmesan cheese, divided into two ¼ cups
1 teaspoon salt
¼ teaspoon pepper

2 cups chopped fresh broccoli
1 and ½ cups julienne carrots
1 cup diced onion
1 fifteen-ounce can diced tomatoes, well-drained
1 or 2 garlic cloves, minced
2 teaspoons vegetable oil

2 cups small-curd cottage cheese
1 cup (4 ounces) shredded mozzarella cheese
½ cup shredded Swiss cheese
1 teaspoon dried oregano

12 lasagna noodles, cooked and drained

½ cup shredded cheddar cheese

In a heavy saucepan, melt butter and add flour. Cook until mixture bubbles. Add milk slowly and stir into a smooth sauce. Reduce heat; add one fourth cup of the Parmesan cheese, salt, and pepper. Cook one minute longer or until cheese is melted. Remove from heat; stir in spinach. Set one and one half cup of this sauce aside.

In a large skillet, sauté the broccoli, carrots, onion, and garlic in oil until crisp-tender. Remove from the heat and add the diced tomatoes; set aside.

In a bowl, combine the cottage cheese, mozzarella, Swiss cheese, and oregano.

Spread three-fourth cup of spinach mixture in a greased ten-by-fourteen-by-two-inch baking dish. Layer with four noodles, half of the cheese mixture, half of the vegetables, and three-fourth cup of the spinach mixture. Repeat layers. Top with remaining noodles, reserved spinach mixture, and reserved Parmesan.

Cover. Bake at 375 degrees for thirty-five minutes. Uncover. Bake for fifteen minutes longer or until bubbly. Remove from oven; sprinkle top with cheddar cheese. Let stand for fifteen minutes before serving. Yield: twelve servings.

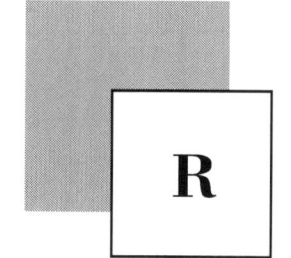

R \\'är\\ (also r)
n. (pl. rs or r's)
the eighteenth letter of the alphabet

ROSES

Recipe: Candied Rose Petals

Recipe: Rose Petal Tea

Recipe: Rose Petal Potpourri

ROSES

"There are tiny buds on the roses," Jay said one warm April afternoon, a mix of anticipation and elation in his voice. The year was 2011, the spring of our fiftieth wedding anniversary.

His love for roses had not yet bloomed when I first met him in the 1950s. He was a college senior, an editor of the yearbook, and looking for someone to write a paragraph to accompany the group picture of my high school freshman class. He tells me my subject-verb agreement impressed him! What impressed me were his blue eyes and being noticed by a college guy!

After his graduation, he left for Cleveland, Ohio, where he satisfied his alternative service requirement by working as a records clerk in a university hospital and where he began studies for a master's degree in English at Case-Western Reserve University. I saw him once briefly—the summer after my sophomore year—at Laurelville, when he made a brief stop during my week at Teen Camp. He remembered me!

Mr. Landis showed up again in the fall of 1956, employed as a high school teacher at EMC. Fun-loving and still unmarried, he was a favorite teacher; not a few of the girls were in love with him. He seemed to love *all* his students *and* his subject, English, that he taught with glad enthusiasm. He was my teacher for English IV and a speech class called oral expression.

The following summer as he made arrangements for the MYF national conference (Mennonite Youth Fellowship) scheduled to meet on the EMC campus and needed a local person to give the welcome speech at the banquet, I came to mind. He would help me, he promised, and I agreed to do it. His help included several evening visits to our farm where we sat on the porch swing and talked into the evening, our topics ranging far beyond speech making.

Soon after the conference, he stopped by Martin's Store where I was working as a retail clerk and handed me a tiny envelope. The little "thank you" card inside simply said, "Dear Peggy, In appreciation, please accept a supper date out Saturday evening. Sincerely, Jay."

We drove out Route 33 East in Jay's black Ford searching for "The Golden Lantern," a new restaurant reputed to have good seafood but discovered its actual name was "The Copper Kettle!" To us, it made little difference and became our joke for many years, proof that love is blind. Later that evening, Jay made his purpose clear and said if I were willing to stop my two-year relationship with a steady boyfriend, we could begin dating.

I carefully considered my options but not for very long. This son of Lancaster, the Red Rose City, was himself truly a red rose!

And so began the growing friendship and long courtship throughout my four years of college. In January 1960, Jay brought flowers one evening and proposed, but we kept our engagement a secret until June when we let our families know one Sunday afternoon through a Scrabble board arrangement. A few weeks later, we mailed a cryptic note to our friends addressed from 50 Wimpole Street, London, England, home of Elizabeth Barrett Browning, the poetess who wrote "How do I love thee? Let me count the ways."

Later that summer when our European student tour brought several of us back to London for five weeks, Jay and I enjoyed some rainy afternoons in an upstairs sitting room of the London Mennonite Center crafting the first plans for our wedding the following summer.

June 10, 1961, had been mostly sunny with a late afternoon shower that freshened the world. The time was eight o'clock in the evening, this late hour unwisely chosen so that our many candles would make a glowing impression! The place was the EMC chapel auditorium, and the platform was banked with baskets of white gladiola, fern stands, and candelabra. Our brothers, Jim and Mart, and several other ushers had seated more than four hundred guests who waited expectantly in the pews. We had mailed about two hundred invitations bearing their four-cent stamps, but it was essentially an open wedding. We heard about one community woman, whom we hardly knew, that had been invited to a nephew's wedding in Pennsylvania on the same day. Since she was unable to attend that event, she just came to ours!

"Let All the World in Every Corner Sing," sung from the balcony of the chapel by the Vesper Chorus (about fifty high school students directed by Audrey B. Shank), opened the short program of music before the processional. When stanza one of "O Perfect Love" began, members of the wedding party readied for their entrances. Back stage left, the ministers, Harold Eshleman and Ira Miller, checked their Bibles and notes. Groomsmen Jim Hertzler, John Lapp, John Martin, and Paul Thomas secured their boutonnieres; best man Roy Burkholder adjusted his tie.

My attendants waited in the vestibule for their long walk down the center aisle. Maid of honor, Ruth Eshleman (Schrock), and bridesmaids, Charity Shank (Showalter), Mildred Rhodes (Eby), Marlene Collins (Showalter), and Audrey Musser (Murray) wore street-length aqua taffeta gowns with matching lace bolero jackets and carried red carnations.

In the language of flowers, the red rose signifies love and romance, the message my cascade of a dozen red roses and baby's breath intended to convey. I had sewed my own white satin floor-length princess-style gown and its short lace jacket with pointed sleeves and tiny satin buttons. Jay's dark suit had been tailor-made, and he wore a single red rose boutonniere. His coat had no lapels, and my veil was a simple head covering, vestiges of the Mennonite plain clothing era and a requirement for EMC faculty at that time. In our small world, we were dressed well for the occasion.

Our vows were the formal poetry of tradition. When my pastor and mentor for many years, Harold Eshleman, asked, "Wilt thou have this man to be thy husband, and wilt thou pledge thy troth to him in all love and honor, in all duty and service, in all faith and tenderness to live with him and cherish him according to the ordinance of God in the holy bond of marriage?" I answered, "I will."

And when our hands were joined, we each repeated after the minister "to have and to hold from this day forward for better, for worse, for richer, for poorer, in sickness and in health, to love and to cherish till death us do part according to God's holy ordinance; and hereto, I plight thee my troth."

After Ira Miller's warm voice intoned the beautiful prayer of blessing he had written for the occasion, we turned to face our friends, and the joyful "Hosanna, Blessed Is He that Cometh in the Name of the Lord!" from *David, the Shepherd Boy*, burst from the chorus in the balcony.

We fear we strained the patience of our guests as they waited to greet us in the receiving line, but most were there to see us feed each other the first bite of cake and drink our raspberry punch in the assembly room downstairs.

It was late when we climbed into Mart's car for the drive to Dayton where ours was hidden in Granddaddy Suter's garage. No tin cans to worry about, Mart's car had instead been lavishly decked inside with garden roses—the fragrant gift of Vesper Chorus students who wished us well!

It was later still when we crossed the mountain for the first night of our honeymoon in the bridal suite of the Luray Caverns Motel. The proprietor had left a note and a key and had gone to bed. We spent most of the week on the Atlantic City, New Jersey shore where we walked on the boardwalk, tried the as yet very cold waters of the ocean, read Shaw's *Saint Joan* together under a beach umbrella, went to movies, and enjoyed the beach food and restaurants.

Friday evening when we returned to our apartment at 1401 Park Road, we discovered that "guests" had been there in our absence to short-sheet our bed and tape cartoons and clippings on every flat surface! On Saturday, we realized that we needed to lay up provisions for the life ahead, so we went to the Mick-or-Mack grocery to stock our cabinets and refrigerator. The forty-eight items, each costing less than a dollar, rang up to a grand total of $19.71! And so began our married life!

There have been many lovely roses in the years since. A large vase of two-dozen red ones was sent to my hospital room by the ecstatic father of our new baby twin daughters. Some years later, those daughters, Ann and Jill, commissioned poet Jean Janzen to write a poem commemorating our fortieth anniversary. In it, Janzen likens marriage to rose care.

> For wedded love
>
> is loosened into time by those
> who bend and serve each other,
>
> their arcs of giving glowing
> into widening worlds. A marriage
>
> like roses born from winters'
> waiting and the patience of pruning . . .
>
> finding an order for two,
> then four, and more.

Most cherished, perhaps, have been the bouquets of roses Jay has clipped through the years from our own gardens—hybrid tea roses with romantic names like Pink Peace, Sedona, Rio Samba, Snowfire, Burning Desire, and Raspberry Parfait, each a testament of Jay's loving care—that I too have known these fifty years.

Rose petals are edible, and their uses are limited only by one's imagination. Jay's fifty rose bushes produce plenty of petals to play with! It is important, however, that the petals you eat come straight from a garden and are not store-bought in order to be sure that no pesticides or fungicides have been used. Sprinkle fresh petals that have been gently rinsed over salads, omelets, cheese trays, or custard desserts.

Candied Rose Petals were a favorite treat in Victorian times. To make this delicate confection, one needs:

> 24 small colorful well-formed rose petals
> 2 egg whites, slightly beaten
> 1 cup superfine sugar.

Brush both sides of the petals with a thin coating of egg white. Sprinkle both sides lightly with superfine sugar and place on a tray sprinkled with additional sugar. Sift another light cover of sugar over the bare spots and allow to set at room temperature overnight. Use to decorate cakes, petit fours, or as a dessert topping.

Rose Petal Tea is fragrant, has fine flavor, and is a lovely dark pink color. The spice and fruit flavors add character to this herbal tea.

½ cup tightly packed deep pink rose petals
¼ teaspoon ground nutmeg
1 teaspoon sugar
¼ orange, peeled and coarsely chopped
1 quart water

Place rose petals, nutmeg, sugar, and chopped orange into a teapot or pitcher. Pour boiling water over petals and steep for five minutes. Strain. Serve hot or cold.

Rose Petal Potpourri (nonedible!) can find a home anywhere; a fragrant perfume is welcome.

3 cups pink rose petals
3 cups red rose petals
2 cups miniature rosebuds
2 cups lavender
1 cup small rose leaves
Cloves, dried citrus peel, tiny pinecones
(optional, but give nice texture)
2 tablespoons powdered orrisroot or other fixative
15 drops rose oil

1. Spread the fresh petals, rosebuds, lavender, and leaves on a mesh screen or large tray. Place them in a warm, dry place and stir gently every day until they are completely dry. Transfer to a large glass or metal bowl.
2. Add the fixative and rose oil. These are vital elements. The fixative absorbs and retains the scented essences. The oil reinforces the natural perfumes and boosts the scent. Use a ratio of two tablespoons fixative to four cups dried material. Mix gently with your hands.
3. Place in a paper bag and seal the top with clothespins or clips. Turn the bag over several times to distribute the fixative. Store away from sunlight and allow the mix to season for four to six weeks. Gently shake the bag from time to time.

When the potpourri is seasoned, it can be placed in a basket or ceramic dish in a warm place, displayed in a covered apothecary jar, or enclosed in small organza or batiste and lace sachet bags. Add several drops of rose oil and mix gently with your hands as the fragrance diminishes.

Potpourri from petals of the summer rose garden can become fragrant gifts for the winter holiday season with just a little long-range planning!

S

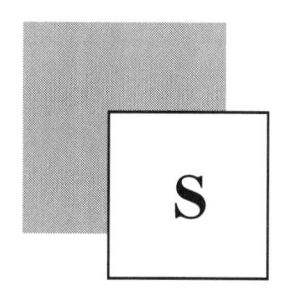

\'es\ (also s)
n. (pl. ss or s's)
the nineteenth letter of the alphabet

SISTERS, SEEKERS, SMALL GROUP

Recipe: Rebecca's Sweet Potato Cranberry Bake

STUDENT

Recipe: Strawberry Shortcake

SISTERS, SEEKERS, SMALL GROUP

"Friends are the family we choose for ourselves."

—Greeting card sentiment

Sisters

My desire for a sister was largely satisfied when I adopted three of them. We four women—we call ourselves the "Wednesday Sisters"—gather in a booth at the local Dairy Queen almost every Wednesday. We have met "to solve the problems of the world" for the last ten or twelve years; we can no longer remember exactly when we took on the challenge!

We do remember the early days of our friendship when, as busy young mothers with careers, we gathered our families under a pavilion on the occasional Saturday morning to cook breakfast in the park. Those were sumptuous meals—grilled ham slices, scrambled eggs, fried potatoes, fresh fruit, and coffee. Once, Naomi even made homemade donuts on location! While our eleven children dabbled in the stream or caught Frisbees, we adults traded news and views and relaxed from our weekday responsibilities.

My oldest "sister" is Irene, cheerful and loving, with sparkling brown eyes. As teachers, she and I drove to school together one year. I left her at the front steps of Dayton Elementary and went on through the back parking lot to Turner Ashby High. In the spring, her third child, Susan, was born and the following fall Ann and Jill arrived. She gave me a baby shower and served strawberry Bavarian pudding in Susan's baby food jars. Irene and Jim were each born in West Virginia and generously share stories about their mountain homes. One day, we four sisters drove the fifty-mile journey to "The Cove," Irene's home near Mathias, where we had lunch in a spotless little diner that served country ham sandwiches and homemade pie. Afterward, we shopped in the general store, admiring the local crafts, wild berry jellies, and staples of all kinds. Generous Irene often gifts us with pints of maple syrup drawn from the trees of the mountain land she still owns.

Naomi's home state is Pennsylvania where she began her long career as an early childhood educator in a country school. From there, she went on to become an advocate for young children and the founder and first teacher in EMU's laboratory program. She is the matriarch of her family, a role imposed on her by the massive stroke John suffered at only forty-two years of age. She is my best example of a "steel magnolia," a strong woman with a gentle, nurturing heart. Tradition matters. Never an Easter morning dawns without a gift of homemade sweet rolls for each of her three children's breakfast tables.

Naomi is the first of our sisterhood to become a great-grandmother. To celebrate LaMya's approaching arrival, we four drove to Staunton to select Beatrix Potter fabric for a crib quilt. It was a joint effort all the way. Irene taught us to appliqué, and we all worked an equal number of squares. After I put the blocks together with sashing and June showed us how to knot a quilt, we completed our project in time for the baby shower.

June was born in Illinois, a twin so tiny she and her sister were kept warm on the oven door. Since those early prairie days, hearth and home have been at the core of her being. We sisters don't need to subscribe to *Better Homes and Gardens* because June is our consultant. Her home is charming, and the plants in her lawn and garden flower and flourish at her touch. She knows them all by name! For many years, it has been June's bright voice and smile that have greeted callers and visitors to EMU. When the day is done and it's too dark to work outside any longer, she and Luke relax with Boston Terrier Daisy and plan the next rendezvous with their family.

When June's mother became critically ill in Illinois one year, she went home for a while to care for her. Our table felt incomplete without June, so each Wednesday when we met for lunch, we passed Irene's cell phone among us to bring her into our circle, if only briefly. It was during this time that significant bonding occurred as we all realized again that life hands out hard experiences, and we all need our friends to carry us through them. Each of us has faced extended caregiving for a father, mother, spouse, child, or grandchild. Around our table, we have an understanding of those challenges.

The years seem to gather momentum since we have crested the hill, but we brake for birthdays and anniversaries! We figure we save so much money eating Kid's Meals and Sweet Deals at Dairy Queen that we can upgrade for birthdays and splurge at downtown eateries. We also save by regifting our gift bags which we fill again with the small items women love—candles, lotions, note cards—simple tokens of our thoughts.

In 2011, we marked the final golden anniversary of our foursome when Jay and I achieved our fifty years. Remarkably, all of our four couples made it to that milestone, and we feted each in turn with a breakfast meal. Jay and I were taken to the grand old Mimslyn in Luray, Virginia, to indulge in the plenteous Sunday brunch and linger over coffee with our friends.

What the Wednesday sisters do best is talk! More than two hours can easily roll by without a pause as we trade concerns about family members, plans for the holidays, impressions of books we have recently read, recipes we recommend, news of department store sales, and compliments on new clothing. We seek each other's wisdom on trivial and important questions—how should we respond to a friend's illness? Where should we live in retirement? Should we buy organic food? Should we treat all adult children the same regardless of their financial circumstances? Where do you go for good medical care? We may sprinkle in a little gossip on occasion, just to keep things spicy, and spontaneous laughter often turns heads in our direction. We know that we can speak in confidence because the years have developed layers of trust that is the foundation of all true friendship.

Seekers

In alphabetical order, the five members of the Seekers group are Marie, Mary, Miriam, Peggy, and Virginia. We Seekers meet monthly in our homes by an alphabetical rotation based on these first names. The hostess selects a short passage of scripture which may be a psalm, a story from the Gospels, a set of verses on a common theme, or another instructive passage, and then makes a copy for each woman in the group. Just before the others arrive, the hostess lights a candle. She prepares no food—this group does not serve refreshments!

After some friendly catch-up, the chosen scripture is read a total of six times, following a modified form of the *lectio divina* (holy reading) structure. Kathleeen Norris, poet, essayist, and oblate in a Benedictine community, says *lectio divina* is a core experience of the Benedictine life, "a daily meditation on scripture in which one reads not for knowledge or information but to enhance one's life of faith." (p. 277) "It is the freedom to ask anything of scripture without requiring an answer or expecting to reach a conclusion, let alone to fit the scripture into one's preconceptions." (p. 279) "Although Benedictines practice *lectio* privately, they are well aware of its communal dimension and the way that *lectio* can instruct a person who wishes to take the Bible personally without privatizing it." (p. 281) (*Amazing Grace*, Riverhead Books, 1998)

In our Seekers' meeting, the first reader thoughtfully reads the chosen passage aloud two times while the others listen for a word or phrase that holds meaning for them. The readings are followed by a time of silence and reflection, after which each person shares the word or phrase from their meditation with the others. This is done without much elaboration.

Then the passage is read two more times, again followed by silence while each woman reflects on how what she has heard touches her life today. These thoughts are also shared with the others.

As the passage is heard two more times, each woman listens for what she believes God is inviting her to do this week. This is followed by sharing at greater length, including requests for prayer. The evening concludes as each woman prays aloud, remembering specifically the requests of the person sitting to her right.

This communal meditation on scripture, with sincere and honest asking for better understanding, and the shared applications to daily experiences open the Bible in amazingly fresh ways. Many times a familiar passage develops from a tight bud to an open flower as we explore its layers of meaning. In the same way, our friendship expands as we open our lives to each other, and we leave spiritually strengthened by this circle of sharing and prayer.

Small Group

If it's the second or fourth Monday of the month, then it's time for "small group!" We have never given ourselves a better name, although one year when our group size was down a little, we called ourselves the "Soup Group." With several empty places around the table, we decided to invite others from church to join us each evening for a supper centered round the soup tureen. In this way, we learned to know some of our church's leaders, new members, and people with recent adventures a little better.

I don't recall that we ever discussed giving our small group a name, although we've discussed just about everything else, but if we happen to consider that possibility sometime, I would like to propose that we call ourselves "The Table Group." Sharing food has been one very consistent activity for our small group of eight.

Another consistent activity has been discussion centered on a book or audio visual series. We gather in the soft and easy chairs of our living rooms and take our turns being discussion leader. Over the years, we have considered materials written or edited by authors such as Kathleen Norris, Anne Lamott, Elizabeth O'Connor, Philip Yancey, Richard Foster, and N. T. Wright.

The host always has the prerogative to take a hiatus from an extended study by announcing a potluck supper or the celebration of a holiday. Once near Mother's Day, each member brought a picture of his or her mother and introduced her to the group. Another evening, we celebrated Columbus Day with a history quiz and the construction of little boats from vegetables and toothpicks. One Halloween, we painted faces of celebrities on pumpkins!

While there may be a certain amount of spontaneity regarding our discussion topic or activity, there is one absolute expectation—dessert! Who would consider the evening complete without gathering around the table to enjoy Ruth's creamy pumpkin cake roll, Hannah's berry cobbler with ice cream, or Shirley's red and white Valentine table displaying cake and ice cream topped with raspberry sauce? Rachel's fruit kuchen carries a hint of her sojourn in Germany, and the season of spring brings on my taste for strawberry rhubarb crunch. I am sure we could compile the many dessert recipes from our dozen or more years into a handsome cookbook!

One cookbook that inspired an interesting dinner for our group is *Mennonite Girls Can Cook* (Schellenberg, et. al., Herald Press, 2011). The book was brand-new when Betty and Lowell gave me and Jay a copy for our fiftieth anniversary. Needing to host the next small group meeting at our house, I selected a menu of recipes all from the new cookbook and set up the dinner event. We too are Mennonite "girls," and we can cook!

The first course included leafy lettuce salad brought by Hannah and Joe, and Ruth baked bubbat (bread) with bits of ham. The main course featured holubschi (cabbage rolls) and mashed potatoes which Jay and I provided. Hannah added glazed carrots for our vegetable side dish. The dessert course included obst moos (cold fruit soup) simmered by Shirley and Kenton, and obst kuchen (blueberry coffee cake) baked by Rachel. To complement the food, Jay selected short readings from the book which led to reflections on the journeys of our German-Russian Mennonite "cousins." Certainly, they can cook and have a long tradition of good food.

Periodically, the group has a planning session about what to do next. One year, Hannah suggested that we "travel" by having each household focus on a place they have visited or would like to visit. Jay and I were first with a preview of our upcoming trip to Russia. We served our guests borscht and blinis before we went to the living room for some Russian trivia and a recent article about the country from a *Time* magazine.

Rachel's PowerPoint presentation and twenty-question quiz pretty well documented the fact that we were all ignorant on the subject of Iceland. Who would have thought that Icelanders drink more Coca-Cola than any country or grow lots of bananas in their greenhouses? For dessert, it was banana pudding with a vanilla sauce and tea.

Kenton and Shirley topped off a review of their recent trip to Australia and New Zealand with Pavlova, a meringue shell with whipped cream and fruit. Joe and Hannah took us to Columbia, South America, and served a mango mousse with pineapple cookies, and Ruth concluded our travels with a video view of Nepal and beautiful platters of cheeses and fresh fruits.

Sometimes the group takes on an evening service project, such as cleaning the wax from many small tapers used at the Christmas Eve candlelight service or helping Kenton prepare little packages of postage stamps for sale at Gift and Thrift. Even a service emphasis can involve food. When a dear friend had cancer, we used the church kitchen to prepare a variety of meals for the family freezer. Each of our five households brought the ingredients for two meals to be prepared and cooked as we worked together. The good-smelling, nutritious-looking soups and casseroles were delivered along with our love and prayers.

The holidays always offer one more opportunity for a party meal, and our small group has never been known to decline the invitation! One year when

Rebecca and Rob were part of the group, we had an especially elegant meal served at our house. Hannah and Joe brought shrimp and cocktail sauce for the appetizer and offered a toast to the health of our group with the wine they also brought.

The main course was served buffet-style and included the German sourdough bread Rachel had baked, oriental spinach salad (Shirley and Kenton), roast chicken (Peggy and Jay), and two vegetable side dishes, yams with cranberries, and baked corn (Rebecca and Rob).

The grand finale was Ruth's beautiful chocolate trifle and coffee. Afterward, we sat in the living room to sing the half-dozen Christmas carols Jay led, a little too full but able to make a joyful noise! As our guests departed, we gave each household a fresh pineapple tied with a red ribbon and Christmas greeting.

Rebecca's yam and cranberry dish was so festive-looking and delicious that several asked for the recipe, which she generously gave. I have used it often, each time remembering our small group friends and the good food we have shared together at each other's tables.

REBECCA'S SWEET POTATO CRANBERRY BAKE

4 large sweet potatoes

2 cups fresh or frozen cranberries
½ cup packed brown sugar
2 tablespoons butter, melted
½ cup orange juice

Topping

½ cup chopped walnuts
¼ cup packed brown sugar
½ teaspoon ground cinnamon
3 tablespoons cold butter

Place sweet potatoes in a pan; cover with water. Bring to a boil. Reduce heat; cover and simmer for forty to fifty minutes or until tender. Drain. When cool enough to handle, peel potatoes and cut into one-half-inch slices.

Place half of the potatoes in a greased two-and-a-half-quart baking dish. Top with half of the cranberries, brown sugar, and butter. Repeat layers. Pour orange juice over all. Cover and bake at 350 degrees for thirty minutes.

In a bowl, combine walnuts, brown sugar, and cinnamon; cut in butter. Sprinkle over the baked dish of sweet potatoes. Return to the oven and bake uncovered for ten minutes or until brown.

Serves six or eight.

STUDENT

There we were in the fall of 1952, perched in our hard wooden desks, twenty-two fledglings recently hatched from elementary schools, hoping to fly through our high school years on the campus of Eastern Mennonite College in Harrisonburg, Virginia.

Properly attired, the thirteen-year-old boys were wearing long sleeves and dress pants. The girls were wearing dresses with sleeves below the elbow and hems four inches below the knee. We had on stockings with seams in the back and the white net prayer coverings on our heads indicated our place in the hierarchy outlined by first Corinthians, chapter eleven. This shade of nonconformity was somewhat darker than I was accustomed to, but I conformed. I pinned up my hair because I wanted to be there with my friends.

The teacher standing at the front of the old Ag Building classroom was Wilmer Landis. He was wearing a severe "plain coat." He had thin blond hair, steel-blue eyes, a reddish complexion, and precise diction.

Our Guidance class used the Book of Proverbs as text, a rich source of maxims to instruct us in our moral development and point us in the way of wisdom. "Which is harder," Brother Landis asked, "to do a daring but dangerous thing some friends are doing or to stand back alone and not take a risk?" We discussed this and other dilemmas before finding the answer in Proverbs. "My son, if sinners entice you, do not give in to them." (Proverbs 1:8 NIV)

Certainly, I was shaped by religious teachings such as this along with the daily chapels I attended for nine long years. I remember very few specifics of those chapel services, but I do remember my teachers, men and women, who walked with us as daily examples of the upright.

Miss Grace Lefever was one of those teachers, a plain red-haired woman who stalked through the classroom and tolerated no nonsense. Indeed, we never put her to the test, so busy we were with her instruction. I was humiliated by my grade on the first general science test and vowed to myself that it would never happen again! And so I studied, and my grades improved. I did learn some science that year, but more importantly, I learned how to study, a skill that stood by me through all my years as a student.

Throughout high school, the English and literature classes were always my favorites. In the freshman year, A. Grace Wenger's radiant smile and warm voice conveyed to us that she genuinely liked us! She was an excellent teacher of writing, practicing affirmation and encouragement to call forth greater efforts from her students. In the sophomore year, dear Arlene Bumbaugh taught *Silas Marner* by George Eliot, the story of a miser whose love for gold was ultimately replaced by his love for Eppie, a golden-haired foundling.

Vivian Beachy taught American literature in the junior year, and I embraced almost everything in the green Harcourt, Brace, and Company book. *Our Town* by Thornton Wilder and the poetry of Sara Teasdale, Emily Dickinson, and others are still among my favorites.

When we returned for our senior year, there was a new teacher on campus. He was Jay B. Landis, twenty-four, and fresh from graduate study in Cleveland, Ohio. Almost immediately, he was everyone's favorite teacher because he was single and fun, and he learned to know us as individuals and became involved in our extracurricular activities as well as our academics. He whetted our interest in such unlikely authors as eighteenth-century Alexander Pope by introductions like asking half a dozen of students what time it was. When all watches disagreed by seconds or more, he revealed:

> *'Tis with our judgments as our watches—none*
> *Go just alike, yet each believes his own.*
> (An Essay on Criticism, Part I, ll. 9-10)

He chilled us with his oral interpretation of the murder of Duncan by Macbeth and entertained us in spare minutes before the bell with *The Education of Hyman Kaplan* by Leonard Q. Ross.

I adored him but had no illusions of romance. He was, after all, older, more experienced, and my teacher. Besides, I was "in love" with my steady boyfriend of two years.

Social activities enriched our high school years. The Massanutten Peak climb in the fall, School Day Out to a secret location in the mountains, Armerian and Philomethean literary societies (I was a Phillie), intramurals, and class trips to Williamsburg and Washington DC encouraged friendships.

Each year, the junior class planned the Junior-Senior Outing, a creative, all-day event with a secret agenda in honor of the senior class about to graduate. I was on the food committee, and our dessert was to be strawberry shortcake. A crew of girls came to my house to bake the hot milk cake. My mother supervised the beating of dozens of eggs and cups of sugar into creamy smoothness. Her later evaluation of the messy process and each girl's competence in the kitchen was based on how well the budding cook handled and scraped the bowl! As I remember, Hazel Knicely, oldest daughter in a large family, would have received Mother's blue ribbon.

The step from the high school (graduation 1957) to the college at Eastern Mennonite was not just across the threshold, even though the campus was the same. It was more like running up a short flight of stairs and arriving breathless at the top! Very quickly, I realized the increased rigors of the academic program.

After giving a little consideration to home economics as my major, I settled on English with enough Latin and education classes to earn a secondary teaching certificate in both disciplines.

I appreciated my college professors, each for his or her best efforts. These deserve special mention: Ruth Brackbill (English), J. Lester Brubaker (Education), Dorothy Kemrer (Latin), Catherine Mumaw (Art Appreciation), Laban Peachey (Psychology), and Hubert Pellman (English).

I was privileged to have Professor Irvin B. Horst for four classes before he left to hold the chair of Church History at the University of Amsterdam. By this time, the early breezes of the Civil Rights Movement of the 60s were beginning to flutter leaves on the EMC campus, precipitating changes at many levels. Professor Horst personified this awakening. He was the quintessential professor-scholar, slightly remote, immersed in his disciplines but kindly aware of his students and their growing restlessness. His opening words in one of our daily chapel talks are the only ones I can quote. "Pull your chair up to the edge of a precipice," he startled us by saying, "and I will tell you a story!" He wore the required "plain coat," but his was slouchy and maroon in color. His contemporary literature class introduced us to Ibsen, Faulkner, Camus, Joyce, and more. I wrote a long paper on *Look Homeward, Angel* by Thomas Wolfe. I woke to a new world in Professor Horst's classes.

My extracurricular activities were mostly literary. I wrote radio scripts for WEMC, 91.7, on the FM dial. I joined Scriblerus, became a member of the 1961 *Shenandoah* yearbook staff, coedited the literary magazine, *The Phoenix*, and acted the role of Margot in *The Diary of Anne Frank*, one of EMC's early drama productions.

Being something of a perfectionist, I studied incessantly during those four years, and my transcript says I finished number 13 in a class of eighty-four. No one has ever asked me for this statistic, so I will tell them now. It ought to be good for something! One warm Monday morning in June 1961, I shook President John R. Mumaw's hand and received my Bachelor of Arts degree.

Thirteen years passed before I received my Master of Arts in Education degree from Madison College (now James Madison University). Ten-year-olds Ann and Jill drew pictures under the shade trees lining the campus in front of Wilson Hall as they waited with their daddy for my brief moment on the stage.

My studies at JMU began in 1969 and progressed a class or two during each summer and one a semester while I was teaching. I finished in 1974. Jay encouraged me and typed my papers, for which I am most grateful. I found that having a master's degree, no matter what field of study it represented, was a ticket to career advancement.

Jay also waited on a wooden bench in the hall while I sat for my comprehensive oral examination. My committee was composed of my major professor, Dr. Jesse Liles, another Education Department professor, Dr. Tony Graham, and my favorite English professor with whom I had taken three language classes, Dr. Lawrence Foley.

Since 1974, I have studied at JMU, EMU, Idaho State University, University of London, and Blue Ridge Community College. Some of these classes renewed my teaching certificate, some supported my work in student services, and many were just for enjoyment. Actually, I have always loved being a student!

STRAWBERRY SHORTCAKE

Mother's Hot Milk Cake

4 eggs
2 cups sugar
2 cups all-purpose flour
2 teaspoons baking powder
1 cup milk
¼ cup butter
1 teaspoon vanilla

1. Beat eggs and sugar with an electric mixer until smooth and pale in color.
2. Sift flour and baking powder together and add to the eggs.
3. Heat milk and butter in a small saucepan until almost boiling. Add slowly to the flour mixture. Add vanilla.
4. Pour into two greased nine-inch round pans or one nine-by-thirteen-inch pan.
5. Bake at 350 degrees for twenty-five to thirty minutes.

Strawberries and Cream

1 and ½ to 2 quarts fresh strawberries
2 tablespoons sugar
Whipping cream or ice cream

Just before serving, cut cake into serving sized pieces and cut each slice into half horizontally. Combine strawberries and sugar. Spoon strawberries between the cake layers and over the top of each serving. Top with whipped cream or ice cream. Garnish with fresh mint leaves, if desired.

This basic yellow cake makes an excellent strawberry shortcake but can be used in numerous variations such as fresh coconut cake or spice cake with caramel icing.

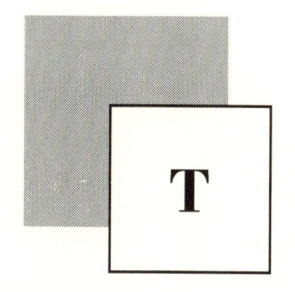

T \'tē\ (also t)
n. (pl. ts or t's)
the twentieth letter of the alphabet

THIMBLE COLLECTION

Recipe: Thimbleberry Pie

TWINS

Recipe: Corn Pudding

Recipe: Savory Squash Bake

THIMBLE COLLECTION

Grandma Landis's pretty silver thimble gives a glimpse into the history of sewing tools in America through a tiny window in the life of Emma Jane (Sheaffer) Landis (1887-1962).

The trademark in the apex of her thimble, MKD, establishes that it was manufactured by the Ketcham and McDougall Company in Brooklyn, New York, sometime between the trademark's introduction in August 1892 and 1932 when the firm stopped making thimbles.

The word *Sterling*, also in the apex, certifies that the thimble contains 925 parts silver out of one thousand. This standard for sterling was established by an act of Congress, and the word has been printed in silver thimbles in the United States since the 1860s.

Grandma's thimble is size 10, considered a medium finger size. There is a wide band above the rim engraved with ten panels, five plain and five decorated with an ornate feather design. The initials "EJS," one letter on each of three of the plain panels, reveal that Grandma received her thimble while she was still unmarried. Proper etiquette at that time did not permit a young man to give his lady any gift that was too personal, such as jewelry or clothing. Flowers, books, or sweets were considered proper gifts, and a fancy gold or silver thimble, engraved with a name or initials, was a most welcome gift. It is possible that her beau, Martin Landis, gave her this pretty thimble, assuring that her thoughts would turn to him whenever she sewed.

Today, Grandma's once gleaming new thimble glows more softly with age, and the indentations around the edge of the cap are almost smooth. Fancy needlework was considered parlor or social activity in those days, and often, the more ornate sewing tools were reserved for embroidery or sewing circle groups, but Grandma's slightly oval, well-worn thimble is evidence that hers was in more frequent use as she sewed her own dresses and mended the family's clothes.

When Grandma Landis died in 1962, Jay's mother gave the thimble to me because she knew I enjoyed sewing. I kept the little treasure for about twenty years before it dawned on me that I had the beginning of a collection!

The first thimble purchase I recall was made in the month of August, sometime in the late 1970s, when Jay and I selected my birthday present from an antiques dealer at the Virginia Highlands Festival in Abingdon, Virginia. It was a good beginning, a sterling thimble with a gold-plated band decorated with ten panels of alternating plain and floral design. This thimble was manufactured by Goldsmith, Stern, and Company sometime between 1913 when the company was founded and 1933 when the business shut down, following the 1929 stock market crash. I didn't know any of that at the time; I chose the thimble from a case simply because I thought it was the prettiest.

A number of years of rather indiscriminate collecting followed. If I saw a sterling silver thimble that I liked at a price I could afford, I bought it. These were also the years when I acquired numerous little brass "work horses," plastic and aluminum advertising thimbles, novelty porcelain, and souvenir thimbles. I subscribed to Franklin Porcelain and purchased three limited editions: *The Butterflies of America* (fifty thimbles, one for each state, 1979); *Thimbles of the World's Great Porcelain Houses* (twenty-five thimbles, 1980); and *The American Heirloom Quilt Thimbles* (twenty-five thimbles, 1984). In retrospect, I defend these purchases. I found all of these thimbles delightful, and I learned a lot in the process.

In 1998 when the silver thimbles alone were numbering about one hundred, I realized how important it was to catalog the collection. I numbered each thimble and logged it into my loose leaf notebook along with a description, size, engravings, and manufacturers' marks. In most cases, I was unable to remember exactly where and when it was bought or the exact cost. Now as the silver collection approaches three hundred, I am amazed by how frequently I consult my log for all these details.

The collection includes a few premium silver thimbles. One I purchased quite by accident at the Harrisonburg Rotary Antique Show for thirty-five dollars from a vender who was as clueless as I was. Imagine my amazement when I discovered "Stitch in Time Saves Nine" in one of my trade books, listed at a value of four hundred fifty dollars! This thimble was known to sell as high as seven hundred dollars in the 1980s and 1990s, but currently, the market has dropped considerably. "Stitch in Time" was made by the Simons Brothers Company established in 1839 in Philadelphia and is currently the only thimble company in America. Simons thimbles are marked with a Gothic "S" inside an upturned bell or shield.

Simons Brothers Company also holds the design patented November 21, 1905, for the applied "Cherubs and Garlands" thimble, sometimes valued as high as three hundred twenty-five dollars. I have two of these thimbles that I was able to purchase for considerably less.

Commemorative thimbles, such as those offered for sale at World's Fair events, are rare finds. The Chicago Columbian Exposition was scheduled to open in 1892 in celebration of the four hundredth anniversary of Columbus's landing in America, but construction problems delayed the opening for one year. The Simons Company sold thimbles using dies with the 1892 date because the production had been started before the announcement of the date change. I found and bought one of these in the Pocono Mountains of Pennsylvania in 1999; around its band are the words, "World's Columbian Exposition 1492-1892."

Several trips to Great Britain presented opportunities to add numerous thimbles to my collection. Delicate bone china souvenir thimbles recall visits to places such as Hampton Court Palace, Shakespeare's birthplace, Cambridge and Oxford, Durham Cathedral, the Bronte Parsonage, and many more. Silver thimbles from the antique markets carry the English hallmarks. Small symbols on the band reveal the first and last initial of the maker, the location of the assay office (the most common being London's leopard's head, Birmingham's anchor, Chester's three corn sheaves, and Sheffield's crown), the Lion passant (the mark for 925 parts fine silver), and the date letter when the thimble was manufactured. In England, one can often find embroidery thimbles—those with an elaborate overall design on the sides and cap.

Charles Horner received his first patent for the Dorcas thimble in England in 1884. Horner stated, "My invention aims to produce a thimble which shall have the appearance of being made of a precious metal and shall be durable and as free of danger of puncturing as though made of steel." This was accomplished by making a thimble with a steel core with outer and inner layers of silver or gold. These thimbles do not carry the assay markings because they are not solid silver but are of such beauty and quality that they rightfully belong in a silver collection. They are marked with "CH" for the maker, the size number, and the name "DORCAS" after the Biblical seamstress who lived outside of Jerusalem at the port of Joppa. Several Dorcas thimbles sit in my cases.

My collection began with a gift and has been enhanced all along the way with gifts. In 1996, Jay's Aunt Naomi gave up sewing and sent me her beautiful silver thimble with a pattern of raised vines known as "Grape," patented by Simons Brothers in 1907 with a listed value of one hundred fifty dollars. On the cartouche are her initials, "NRM." Other gifts include the scrimshaw etched with a whaling vessel from Ellen, the delicate silver in its velvet envelope from Margaret's visit to India, the Williamsburg pineapple from Erma, the beaded bird's head from Lee's trip to China, the sterling thimble with a cut-out border design that once belonged to Lynn's Midwest, minister's wife grandmother.

Many of my thimbles have the initials or the name of the original owner engraved on the band, lovely old names of late nineteenth century women—Ella, Ada, Nettie, Lillian, Clara, Nellie, Lina. Each of these thimbles has lived another earlier life and would have a story to tell. All have worked hard and traveled far; they deserve their rest in my thimble case and the admiration they receive from me and others.

My most cherished thimble is fourteen-karat gold made by Simons Brothers and decorated with the Greek key around the band. It is size 10 and fits my finger. It is engraved with my name, an anniversary gift from Jay, who has supported and supplemented my collection many times, many ways.

Merriam-Webster's *Collegiate Dictionary* defines "thimbleberry" as any of several American raspberries or blackberries (esp. *Rubus occidentalis, Rubus parviflorus,* and *Rubus odoratus*) having thimble-shaped fruit.

Make this delicious Thimbleberry Pie which serves eight people. Enjoy more than a thimbleful!

THIMBLEBERRY PIE

Filling
⅓ cup cornstarch
2 sixteen-ounce cans thimbleberries (blackberries or raspberries), drained, juice reserved
⅓ cup sugar
1 teaspoon finely grated orange zest

Blend the cornstarch with a small amount of the reserved berry juice in a small bowl until smooth.

Combine the remaining juice, sugar, orange zest, and the cornstarch mixture in a small saucepan. Stir over medium heat until the mixture boils and thickens. Remove pan from heat and set aside to cool.

Pastry
2 cups unbleached, all-purpose flour
2 teaspoons sugar
1 teaspoon salt
¾ cup good solid shortening
2 teaspoons vinegar
1 egg, lightly beaten
3 tablespoons water

Mix flour, sugar, and salt. Cut in shortening with pastry blender until mixture resembles cornmeal.

Beat together vinegar, egg, and water. Add to crumb mixture. Combine with fork until all ingredients are moistened.

Turn onto a well-floured surface and knead slightly until dough is smooth. Divide dough, keeping one part slightly larger. Roll the larger part into a circle to fit the bottom of a nine-inch pie plate. Roll the remaining pastry into a circle large enough to cover the top of the pie.

Assembly

Arrange the larger pastry circle in the nine-inch pie plate.

Spread cooled cornstarch mixture evenly into pie shell. Top with the reserved berries.

Spread one tablespoon soft butter lightly over the smaller pastry circle. Decorate as desired, making several small slashes in the dough to serve as air vents. Moisten edges of large circle with water to seal before placing the smaller circle on the plate to cover the berries.

Trim edges of both crusts with a sharp knife. Crimp edges with a fork or fingers. Sprinkle top crust with one tablespoon sugar.

Bake in preheated oven at 400 degrees for ten minutes. Reduce heat to 350 degrees for twenty-five to thirty minutes or until pastry is crisp and golden.

TWINS!

> *Forget that you are now a statistic. Settle down with those two incredible creatures, unlike any other two in the world—as a matter of fact, unlike each other—and prepare yourself for a year of hard work and a lifetime of unalloyed joy, for almost the only concrete, undisputed, unarguable, self-evident fact that everyone agrees upon (experts included) is that some women go to the hospital to have one baby and go home with two.*
>
> Holland-Gehman, *Twins: Twice the Trouble, Twice the Fun*, Lippincott, 1965, p.45.

The sounds I heard in the operating room at Rockingham Memorial Hospital about ten forty on the evening of November 5, 1963, will be forever alive in my mind—the most significant sounds of my life. There were several gasps for breath as little lungs filled and then a vigorous cry. "It's a little girl!" Dr. Eshleman told me with awe in his voice, for when is new life not a miracle? A minute later, another baby's search for air preceded an equally robust cry. "It's another little girl!" the doctor announced with joy. "Dr. Eshleman," I needed to know, "are they all right?" "They appear to be," his soft voice assured me. I had just a glimpse of two bloody, slimy newborns with dark hair as their little incubator cart wheeled past my vision and headed for the nursery and their first baths.

More parents are seeing double these days than Jay and I did in 1963. A 2012 report from the Centers for Disease Control shows that the twin birth rate has risen 76 percent since 1980. About one in every thirty newborns has a twin brother or sister. Technology, fertility drugs, and an older child-bearing age for many mothers help to explain this increase. I have not found a comparable birth rate for twins born in 1963, but some place it at about one in eighty-eight births (Holland-Gehman, p. 32). Ann's and Jill's births were significant enough at the time to warrant a small headline in the local newspaper, "Twins at Hospital."

As the hospital window ledge filled with floral arrangements from friends and family, Jay and I felt more and more like celebrities. Cards and gifts followed—two of everything—sweaters, blankets, dresses, engraved feeding spoons, pajama sets, and more, including diaper service, cribs, and a playpen. Word came that my Latin students, who learned that their teacher on maternity leave was now the mother of twins, each wore *two* pink ribbons in celebration.

The babies were almost full term, active, and healthy. They were pink and plump and absolutely beautiful! At birth, Ann weighed five pounds and nine ounces, and Jill weighed an exact six pounds, so neither needed an incubator. One three-hour and one four-hour feeding schedule kept up a busy pace during my hospital stay.

Hospital practices for new mothers were so different fifty years ago. I recuperated in the hospital for ten days following my cesarean section, spending most of the time in bed. Fathers were not permitted in the labor or delivery areas and did not even hold their babies until the day they left the hospital. Hospital bills were different too! A note Jay made at the time listed hospital and obstetrical services, including doctors' fees, not covered by insurance at $155.05—an incomparable bargain!

My mother helped to transport me and the babies home from the hospital and stayed with us for a whole week. Aunt Helen came from Maryland to assist. While Jay and I sometimes rested comfortably, these two fed babies at all hours of the night. We didn't hear from Aunt Helen for more than a week after she returned by bus and joked that she probably fell asleep and didn't wake until she was long past her depot! Jay's mother came the following week and took her turn with the night duty.

Eventually, they all went home, and we were on our own—an occasion for panic were it not for Jay's total commitment to fatherhood. We learned to feed two hungry mouths, hold and comfort two crying babies, change two messy diapers, bathe two squirmy bodies. Somehow, we survived those early months. Jay continued to teach his seniors with assistance from a student teacher. I suppose I kept our apartment and clothing reasonably clean and cooked our meals, but actually it is a blur. We even managed to purchase a home and move into it during that time.

Even though traveling with twin infants across town was a hassle, parents cannot stay homebound forever. In 1963, there were no car seats and no safety regulations. Jay usually drove, and I sat in the passenger seat of our little Ford Falcon holding one baby on my lap and nestling her little sister on the seat beside my left leg. We never took them anywhere while they were infants unless both of us were on board.

When the girls were able to sit up alone, we often went to the grocery store and each pushed a cart providing two safe places to ride. We soon became aware that the grocery store was a place of open season on parents of twins, providing territory for strangers of every ilk to shoot their questions. Noticing that the same questions were asked over and over, we joked about hanging signs on the carts so we could just point to the answer and move on! What follows is a list of these frequently asked questions with the unabridged answers; we never went into this much detail in the cereal aisle—no peppy baby girl would have been willing to sit still that long!

Are they twins?

This question was usually asked by people who were fascinated by the mystery of twin births or who themselves had a twin story they wanted to tell. It was often the opener for other questions to follow.

Did you know you were having twins?

Yes, but only for about fourteen hours! Rather early in my pregnancy, our family doctor, Merle Eshleman, M. D., suggested the possibility of two but was never able to hear two heart beats. There were no ultrasound pictures, only X-rays, that might have been harmful if taken too early. I had an X-ray appointment scheduled, but the babies came before the appointment. When I arrived at the hospital on the morning of November 5, the X-ray picture revealed the exciting truth! Jay rushed out and called his parents who told him to go and buy a second crib! At this point, Dr. Eshleman referred me to Dr. Walter M. Zirkle, a young obstetrician who delivered his first twins by caesarean later that evening. Dr. Eshleman also brought Dr. L. D. Burtner, a pediatrician, on board to care for the babies.

Are there twins in your family?

Yes, lots of them. My great uncles were twins, my aunt had twins, and several cousins had twins. My niece has twins. Jay's grandfather was a twin, and he has nephews and grandnieces who are twins. They say twins are only hereditary on the mother's side as obviously only the mother ovulates. Some say a son may inherit a hyper ovulating gene which he can pass on to a daughter, making it appear that twins skip a generation. I likely inherited that hyper ovulating gene from my father's side of the family. Jill and Ann may have inherited it from both parents.

Are they identical?

Actually, we have never known a definitive answer to this one. Everyone knows there are two basic categories of twins: identical (monozygotic—one egg) and fraternal (dizygotic—two eggs). At the time of Jill and Ann's births, before the days of DNA testing, we were told that the only conclusive test was grafting skin from one child to the other. Knowing just wasn't that important to us! In fact, we preferred to think of them as two distinct individuals, not two copies of the same person, and didn't particularly want to know.

The girls do share physical similarities as well as interests and abilities. They are both female and looked remarkably alike when they were small.

A little white tooth might appear for each baby within days or weeks. Each has a birthmark on her back that resembles one on my back. However, the doctors told me there were two placentas, a sign of fraternal twins. Only fraternal twins are considered hereditary, and given the frequency of twins in my family, it would be coincidental, but not impossible, for me to bear identical twins. Physical appearance is not conclusive. Many fraternal twins bear strong family resemblance, while many identical twins don't look alike because of environmental influences.

How do you tell them apart?

When Ann and Jill were only a few days old, a nurse brought one to me for a feeding. When the baby had eaten, she was returned to the nursery; and a little later, a second baby was brought. I received her into my arms, but had a strong sense that it was the same little one I had just fed. "Oh, no, Mrs. Landis," the nurse assured me, "but I will go and check." In a few minutes, she was back, carrying another baby and confessing that I had been right. This incident was extremely reassuring to me because it confirmed my ability to know my babies apart.

A few years later, Jill and Ann's preschool teacher had a lesson on the words "same" and "different." "Who is here in our circle that looks the same?" she asked. The little children looked around at each other and concluded that no one did. "How about Ann and Jill?" she prompted. "Do they look the same?" "Oh, no," someone responded, "that is Jill, and this is Ann."

Once again, the secret was in knowing the girls as individuals. Being aware of details and caring enough to remember also helped. Later, we combed their hair in different ways as a marker for friends. Basically though, the shape of their faces differed; Jill had a higher forehead, and Ann's face was a little more round.

Do they cry at the same time?

Of course—but not always. The question behind this question is whether twins are a lot of work and whether one person can manage two babies. Not having experience with one baby before these two were born, we had nothing with which to compare; but certainly those parents who have other children, especially toddlers, have a much greater challenge than we did. Even so, I cannot imagine caring for two infants without their loving father often on duty to help.

When babies are hungry, they cry. If I was home alone, I offered them pacifiers—Ann preferred her thumb—while I warmed their bottles. Then I sat on the couch and held one baby in my arm, while the other lay with pillows beside my leg for half the feeding. After burping, I switched the babies' positions, so each received some cuddling along with her milk. It was an imperfect situation, but you do the best you can.

What are their names?

Since the possibility of twins had been suggested, we packed four names into the hospital suitcase—two for girls, two for boys. Jay liked the name "Ann." I had a student named "Ann" whose second name was "Meredith." A pretty combination, I thought. I liked the name "Jill," and so we searched the baby name books for a second name that flowed well with "Jill" and would be as distinctive as "Meredith." We decided on "Ingrid." Ann Meredith and Jill Ingrid.

Some of our grocery store questioners looked disappointed when they heard the names. They don't rhyme and don't even start with the same letter, their looks implied. Frequently, we heard people refer to the girls as Jan and Jill. Many people found it hard to give up on the idea of making twins as much alike as possible—something we strongly opposed.

Do they usually dress alike?

Yes and no. The darling baby gifts came in duplicates, and the girls looked adorable in them. While we were getting used to the whole crazy idea of having two, it was great fun to show them off and would have been impossible to resist the pressure to do just that. I did some sewing for them as toddlers, and it was just easier to attach one collar and not have to change the bobbin thread for the second collar. When we bought clothing, we usually tried to buy similar outfits in different colors. In high school, Jill and Ann made a point of not wearing identical clothing; they just dressed like all the other teen girls in sweaters, shirts, denim skirts, and blue jeans, which was a uniform of sorts.

Is one more outgoing or advanced than the other?

No question was more provoking to me than this one! When one baby daughter happened to look a stranger in the eye and turn on a dimpled smile, while the other little girl studied a bright color in the distance, some intruders would attempt to demonstrate their brilliant ability to discern personality types by asking a variant of this intrusive question. No one would ever ask a mother of singletons to label her children in this way! It was my signal to shut down the conversation. "They take turns being most outgoing and advanced—and we really do need to go!" I might say as I wheeled my baby toward the checkout.

And it was true! They were generally happy and enjoyed socializing, and they accomplished developmental tasks nicely on schedule. Neither child lagged behind the other for long. Ann was pulling herself up and "walking" around the coffee table, giving every evidence that she would be the one to take her first steps. But to our surprise, Jill suddenly stood up and took off. We soon learned never to make predictions.

Do they have their own special twin language?

As teachers of English and Latin, Jay and I enjoyed our front row seats for the "development of language show" being performed daily in our own home. We read lots of books aloud to the girls and shunned baby talk. They moved easily from "Mama" and "Dada" to longer words like "applesauce." At one stage, they did show a little interest in idioglossia (twin-speak) and created several indecipherable nonsense words which we heard them use on occasion. Two of these that we couldn't find in any version of any dictionary were "stringlejenk" and "hamagretchen." A third word we remember was "pottiaka," and although we never knew its exact meaning, the effect was clear. This word was occasionally hurled from one to the other in anger, a strong invective that caused the receiver to wither in disgrace!

An older neighbor who had an "identical" twin sister enjoyed her twin status very much and sometimes told me stories about their uncanny sameness. When she and her sister were young, they worked in a market where they took separate lunch breaks. One would go first to a nearby diner, order, eat, and return to the market, not telling her sister what she had eaten. When the second twin returned, they compared lunch menus and frequently found that they had ordered the same things.

As alike as "two peas in a pod," some would say. Peas. Vegetables. Vegetable recipes. I decided to conduct my own experiment, less scientific than skin grafting or DNA, but more easily carried out in a kitchen. I asked Ann and Jill, without conferring, to each give me a recipe using a vegetable for this chapter. Would they give me recipes using the same vegetable? Even the same recipe?

Their responses leaned toward the fraternal side of the spectrum. Jill gave me her Grandma Heatwole's corn pudding recipe. She freezes corn in the summer, and her family loves this creamy vegetable casserole. Ann gave savory squash bake, a recipe she concocted in her Florida kitchen using summer squash but delicious in any season. Corn and squash—two different vegetables, both yellow and both preparations baked in the oven. There, the comparison ends!

CORN PUDDING

2 tablespoons cornstarch
2 eggs, slightly beaten
1 to 2 tablespoons sugar, according to taste
12 ounce can evaporated milk
14 and ¾ ounce can cream-style corn or 1 pint home frozen corn
¼ cup cracker crumbs
2 tablespoons melted butter

Mix together cornstarch, eggs, and sugar until smooth.
Add milk, corn, and crumbs.
Pour into greased one and a half quart baking dish. Pour melted butter over top.
Bake in 350 degrees oven for forty-five minutes or until firm in the center.
Makes four to six servings.

SAVORY SQUASH BAKE

2 and ½ lbs. yellow squash
12 ounces reduced-fat bulk sausage
⅓ cup chopped onion

Slice squash into half-inch thick quartered pieces. Steam until tender but still firm (approximately ten minutes); drain. Meanwhile, brown sausage and onion in skillet; drain off excess fat.

½ cup crushed Roasted Vegetable Ritz crackers (or other buttery cracker)
½ cup shredded Parmesan cheese
2 slightly beaten eggs
⅛ teaspoon dried thyme
2 tablespoons dried parsley flakes
Salt and pepper to taste

In a large bowl, mix together sausage, onion, squash, eggs, crackers, cheese, and seasonings. Pour into a two-quart casserole dish coated with vegetable spray.

Topping
1 cup crumbled crackers
¼ cup butter, melted
2 tablespoons shredded Parmesan cheese

Sprinkle mixture and cheese over top of casserole. Bake at 350 degrees for thirty-five to forty minutes. Midway, cover casserole lightly with foil so topping does not burn. Makes six servings.

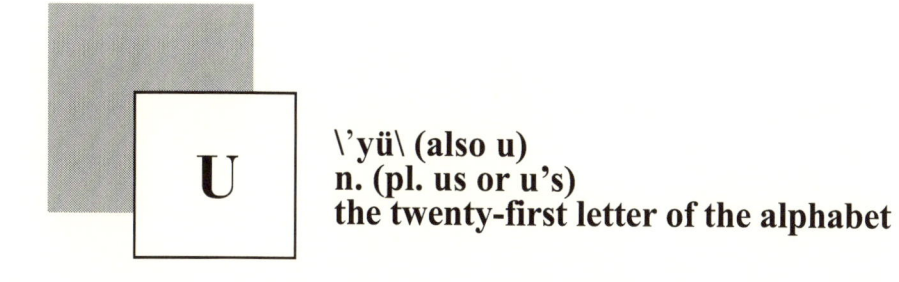

U \'yü\ (also u)
n. (pl. us or u's)
the twenty-first letter of the alphabet

UNCLES, AUNTS, AND COUSINS

Recipe: Aunt Alice's Old-Fashioned Sugar Cookies

UNCLES, AUNTS, AND COUSINS

> *This certainly is a beautiful place. It's up on a hilltop—a windy hilltop—lots of sky, lots of clouds, often lots of sun and moon and stars. . . . Yes, beautiful spot up here. Mountain laurel and li-lacks. I often wonder why people like to be buried in Woodlawn and Brooklyn when they might pass the same time up here. . . . Yes, an awful lot of sorrow has sort of quieted down up here. People just wild with grief have brought their relatives up to this hill. . . . A lot of thoughts come up here, night and day, but there's no post office.*
>
> —Act III, *Our Town*, Thornton Wilder, Coward-McCann Inc., 1938

One morning in 2007, a procession formed at the Mossy Creek Presbyterian Church. Men carried a casket to the "windy hilltop" of the church cemetery, and the people moved forward slowly to stand around a grave overlooking the Virginia "range on range of hills," already pink and green with the promise of spring.

One could almost hear Mrs. Soames from Act III of *Our Town* say, "Who is it, Julia?" But from the adjacent grave, John Patterson gave the answer speaking softly without raising his eyes. "It's my wife, Wilda Heatwole." I stood among the mourners for my aunt and remembered Grover's Corners and the Stage Manager's words. "And we're coming up here ourselves when our fit's over." We were glad Aunt Wilda was in a beautiful place.

Actually, the funeral processions for my father and mother's siblings began much earlier with the untimely deaths of two sisters on two consecutive days during the epidemic of Spanish influenza in 1919. Anna Elizabeth Heatwole, age twenty-one, and Mary Margaret Heatwole, age eighteen, were buried side by side in Weaver's Mennonite Cemetery, their graves marked by a single, tall, ornate headstone erected by my grandfather, distraught with grief. My three-year-old father, also sick with the flu, did not really remember his older sisters who died twenty years before I was born. The scourge that snatched away their lives also robbed us all of personal relationships and memories.

Aunt Edith Heatwole Swope left us in 1957. I was a senior in high school, and her death brought me the horrible realization that mothers can die. My younger cousin Ellen, with whom I had played dolls and stayed overnight, was only fourteen when they picked her up at school one day to begin the time of mourning for her mother. Aunt Edith's illness brought the terrifying word "cancer" into our immediate vocabularies. When she called my mother, her sister-in-law, to her bedside to say goodbye, she told Mother that she had always loved Mother like a sister, words my mother remembered and treasured throughout her life. Aunt Edith's young adult sons, Richard and Roy, walked with Uncle Frank and Ellen in the somber procession to her grassy plot in the Cook's Creek Presbyterian Cemetery, another beautiful place.

Uncle Owen Heatwole was twenty years older than my father and was married the same year Daddy was born. My oldest cousin Charlotte was a year older than my mother. Uncle Owen and Aunt Virgie's youngest daughter Jane was four years my senior but allowed me to play with the dolls she had all but outgrown whenever we went for a Sunday afternoon visit. Uncle Owen was a foreman with the feed division of the Rockingham Cooperative Farm Bureau where Daddy shopped for farm supplies. His death came unexpectedly at the age of sixty-six, one of too many Heatwole men to die too young of a heart attack. His son and my cousin Dwight died of a heart attack when he was fifty-two. Jay and I had been married only several months when we attended Uncle Owen's service at the over-crowded Garber's Church of the Brethren and then followed the funeral car to inter his body several feet away from his parents' grave in the Weaver's Mennonite Cemetery.

The youngest brother's procession followed the oldest brother's procession to the Weaver's Cemetery. Uncle George Heatwole died in 1975, another victim of a sudden heart attack. Only fifty-eight years old at the time of his death, he was active as a farmer and auctioneer and was in his eleventh year as Rockingham County supervisor of the Central District. When I see the peanut oil lamp on my bedroom shelf, I am reminded of how witty Uncle George was as an auctioneer and how pleased he seemed to knock off that lamp to us at Great Aunt Maude's sale! We were in Idaho when Mother's call came early in April. I remember how shocked and sad I felt that day. Mother and Aunt Hazel were best friends from childhood; she died at age eighty-nine in 2006, just eight months after Uncle George and Aunt Hazel's son Paul died unexpectedly—also from a heart attack.

Uncle Earl Heatwole's funeral procession traveled from the Mill Creek Church of the Brethren to another "windy hilltop" in the Keezletown Cemetery in 1981. When he and Daddy both owned farms in the Keezletown vicinity they traded labor, and Jim and I played with cousins Beverly and Linda. A humorous, congenial man, Uncle Earl would joke, "Come on over! We'll plug a huckleberry!" Later when the work was done, we would "plug" a watermelon and spit the seeds in their back yard.

In 2003, Uncle Harold Suter died, the first of Mother's siblings. He was a rotund man with a nice chuckle; Aunt Zettie called him "Pud." I liked to tease him and called him "Herald Angel." He loved everything automotive and operated a repair shop next to their home near Dayton. Later, he was employed as a mechanic with Rockingham County Schools, keeping the fleet of yellow school buses up and running. He liked cars and driving them too. "Making time" and getting places ahead of schedule were his delight. Several times our family and theirs (nine in all) crowded into his well-oiled vehicle for the trip through Washington DC and into Maryland to visit Aunt Helen and her family. Once on our return, we took a wide swing to cross the Chesapeake Bay on a ferry boat, stay overnight in a motel, and eat in restaurants—big time vacation in those days! My cousins Winston, Charlie, and Lonnie, along with Jim and me, played H-O-R-S-E and other basketball games on the floor of their old barn. Sometimes when they came to our house, Mother boiled molasses, and we pulled taffy. Uncle Harold died at age eighty-eight from a rare blood disease called histoplasmosis. After the funeral service in the Dayton United Methodist Church, his body was laid in the Dayton cemetery nearby.

It was July 2004 when we gathered by Aunt Alice Heatwole Suter's grave on another "windy hillside" in another beautiful country cemetery near the Beaver Creek Church of the Brethren. Aunt Alice was ninety-five when she died and still beautiful. I admired her sense of style, stately composure, and beautiful wave of snow-white hair. Was she actually taller than the rest of the women in the room, or did she just seem so to me? She liked nice clothing and when my older cousins, Shirley and Janet, handed down a bag of wool plaid skirts and soft sweaters they had outgrown, I was thrilled! Aunt Alice served bountiful company dinners, magazine picture perfect, but it will be her inimitable iced tea that I'll always remember best. She enjoyed reading and encouraged that pleasure for others. She often gave books to the children at the Heatwole family Christmas gathering, and I still have my *Heidi*, now quite yellow with age.

In 2007, the last of my father's siblings passed away, and it was Aunt Wilda Heatwole Patterson's graveside service at Mossy Creek that brought the fictional cemetery of Grover's Corners to my mind. Aunt Wilda was ninety-five years old, a quiet, kind woman who worked hard alongside her husband John. She loved to work, and even in her last years, my cousin Mary Ellen was challenged to keep her hands busy folding laundry, snapping beans, whatever she could find to make her mother feel useful. Aunt Wilda was the only one of her family to graduate from high school, riding a horse several miles every day to become the valedictorian of her class in 1929. Her platter of country ham was the best at the family reunion. For a wedding gift, she gave us a lovely lace tablecloth, my reminder of her outstanding skills as cook and hostess. When Aunt Wilda's memorial service was concluded, we were all invited to lunch in the church social hall. This traditional conclusion to the funeral ritual was observed at the passing of all my aunts and uncles. My journal says the ladies of the Mossy Creek Presbyterian church served a substantial meal with two meats, macaroni and cheese, several side dishes, and homemade desserts.

My last and dearest aunt left us in 2008, Mother's older sister, Helen Suter Thurman Boyer. Aunt Helen left the valley in her late teens to become a nanny for a family in Washington DC. There, she met debonair Hayward Thurman and produced five sons and a daughter. She was always more than a match for her five prankster sons who thought up outlandish antics to tease her. One night, they scotch-taped the refrigerator door shut, so their petite little mother would wonder why the door wouldn't open when she came to make breakfast in the morning. They knew she would always win in the end—after all, who made the breakfast? In some ways, her distance from the Valley enriched our lives; it provided us a location for overnight visits as children that gave an exposure to the city and a somewhat different culture. After Uncle Hayward's death, an almost forgotten former flame, Charles Boyer, rang her doorbell one night, and the fire was rekindled, a romance for the story books! When Mother was in the nursing home and no longer able to join Aunt Helen in long telephone conversations, Aunt Helen called me instead, and I enjoyed her laughter and chatter for an hour or more. Her gravesite is beside Uncle Hayward's in the Spencerville Cemetery, about a mile from her Free Methodist Church in Maryland.

I still have one uncle! Uncle J. Richard Suter is Mother's youngest brother and lives with Aunt Elizabeth in Charlottesville, Virginia, about an hour from us. Born in 1925, he was only fourteen when I was born; and throughout my childhood, he kept a playful spirit, enjoying all his nieces and nephews. Pretty much a "self-taught" man, his hobbies and interests spilled over to broaden our lives. He taught himself to play the guitar and mandolin. He taught us all to play Rook, long the family's favorite table game. When he took an interest in photography and bought a camera, spotlights, and all, he arranged an appointment with me and set up a "studio" in our dining room where I sat in various poses for my portrait and his practice. One of our first radios was one he built from scratch, but Gene Autry and Roy Rogers came in loud and clear. This hobby turned into a career when he went to work repairing radios and televisions for Magnavox until his retirement. Now we use e-mail and telephone to share titles of books we are reading. He never forgets my birthday. He is all the more special to me because he is my last connection with my parents and grandparents' generation.

These nine families produced thirty-four cousins who lived past infancy. I regret that in comparison, my grandchildren have three families and two cousins. Today, smaller family size and increased mobility of the members take away much of the warmth of the large extended family of my childhood.

Virginia country graveyards are beautiful places, usually well-tended gardens of strong, silent stones, the older ones bleached white, sometimes with names hardly visible. These stones reduce the minute details of many years to a few words and dates, and yet they stand to proclaim that *"something is eternal"* as the stage manager of *Our Town* told us. A few years ago, Jay and I chose plots that look eastward to the Massanutten Mountain from the Weaver's Cemetery. We ordered a single stone which is now in place with all the engraving except the final dates.

Very near our stone stand the stones of Paul W. Heatwole, my first cousin, and Harold Eugene Huber, Jay's first cousin, and other friends we know or have known. Will we talk in soft emotionless tones as they did in the cemetery of Grover's Corners? If so, I will thank Paul one last time for teaching me how to ride a bicycle one Sunday afternoon when we were children at Grandma's house.

One December some years ago, Mother, my sister-in-law Ruby, and I put our four children in the car and drove to Spring Creek for an afternoon visit with Aunt Alice. She was already into her Christmas baking and brought out old-fashioned sugar cookies to serve with her tea. Creamy white with delicate brown edges, her buttery cutouts simply melted away in our mouths. Ruby called and begged the recipe, then shared a copy with me.

AUNT ALICE'S OLD-FASHIONED SUGAR COOKIES

2 cups sugar
1 cup butter
5 eggs
2 teaspoons vanilla extract
3 teaspoons soda
5 and ½ cups flour (or enough to handle well)
1 cup sour cream
Colored sugar sprinkles (optional)

In a large mixing bowl, cream butter and sugar until light and fluffy. Beat in eggs. Add soda and vanilla. Sift flour and add alternately with the sour cream. Cover dough and refrigerate overnight.

Divide dough into fourths. Roll each portion to one-fourth-inch thickness and cut into desired shapes. Place on ungreased baking sheet. Add colored sprinkles before baking, if desired. Bake at 350 degrees for seven to eight minutes or until edges show a light brown. Do not over bake. Remove to wire rack to cool. Yield: eight or nine dozens of cookies.

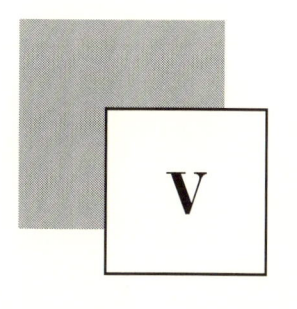

V \\'vē\\ (also v)
n. (pl. vs or v's)
the twenty-second letter of the alphabet

VOLUNTEER

Recipe: Zucchini Egg Foo Yung

VOLUNTEER

My 2001 Journal records two views of retirement on June 20, several weeks before my last day of paid employment. Ray stopped at my office, and I learned that he had retired the previous year; he said retirement was wonderful! When he asked whether I was going to take Social Security early, I asked his advice. "Take it," he firmly recommended. Later that day, my neighbor Diane called to check about block party dates. When she learned that I was soon retiring, she shared that she had stopped work about a year before and missed it so much that she was thinking of going back. She missed getting up and getting going in the morning.

Interestingly, I had read a story in Luke 12 that very morning that seemed to apply. Most people in the first century AD didn't have the option of working or not working, but they did have questions about wealth and inheritance. To one of these, Jesus responded with the parable of the rich man who tore down his barns to build bigger ones. This rich man said to himself, "You have plenty of good things laid up for many years. Take life easy; eat, drink, and be merry." With this story, Jesus warned his listeners to guard against greed, saying, "A man's life does not consist in the abundance of his possessions." This may be as close as Jesus came to talking about the questions of modern-day retirement: What shall I do with my time? What shall I do with my accumulated possessions?

Reflecting on the past twelve years of my retirement, I realize that I have been a regular part-time worker for Mennonite Central Committee (MCC). The CEOs in the head offices in Akron, Pennsylvania, don't send a paycheck; in fact, they don't even know my name. I am a volunteer, one of over ten thousand in the United States and Canada who work for MCC.

The MCC organization began in 1920 after World War I when representatives from various church conferences formed a committee and pledged to aid hungry people, including many Mennonites in Russia and the Ukraine. Now MCC has workers or financial commitments in more than fifty countries around the world. The work is concrete and hands-on, addressing basic human needs such as water, food, shelter, education, health, and peace building, all in the name of Christ. MCC's priorities are disaster relief, sustainable community development, justice, and peace building. Programs cross cultural, political, and economic divides. This is the kind of work I can happily support with my time and money.

Thousands of volunteers across the United States and Canada help MCC by donating time and money. Those who cannot work in full-time assignments assist by volunteering in thrift shops and fair trade outlets, relief sale efforts, and meat canning operations. Others assemble kits for humanitarian aid, sew comforter blankets, and participate in advocacy campaigns.

Shortly after I closed the door of my office for the last time, I received a call from my friend Nancy, president of the local Gift and Thrift, 227 North Main Street in Harrisonburg. This shop is one of a network of MCC shops that now numbers 113 in Canada and the United States, generating contributions totaling $167 million during the forty years since the first shop began in 1972. "Thrift" contributes to the worldwide relief efforts of MCC through the sale of donated items, and "Gift" assists international artisans and farmers in developing countries by marketing their fairly traded products.

The September 4, 2001, entry in my journal reports on my first day of work. "The new thing today was my afternoon at the Gift and Thrift store as a volunteer cashier. Deb Layman is the comanager with husband Ken. She is such a capable woman, has things so well organized, and manages about eighty volunteers in sorting, pricing, displaying, sales, and furniture repair. She showed me how to operate the cash register that isn't hard if you're careful—it even figures the sales tax automatically! I was surprised at the number of shoppers, not a rush but a steady coming and going all the time. Receipts at the end of the day totaled over seven hundred dollars, and that came from items priced from ten cents to ten dollars. (I sold only one ten-dollar item.)"

In 2004, Gift and Thrift moved to the 28,000 square foot, completely renovated Ray Carr Tire building at 731 Mount Clinton Pike and included three divisions—Thrift, Gift, and Booksavers, a new book operation consisting of retail and Internet sales and a small paper baling process. I moved with the Thrift operation, still working as a cashier.

A year later when Deb and Ken opened a second thrift shop, Tried and True on the east side of Harrisonburg, a small shop with a boutique appearance, I followed Deb to the new store. Tried and True is also a nonprofit that benefits MCC, specifically the Generations-at-Risk program for HIV/AIDS care and prevention in Africa.

In 2009, Gift and Thrift completed a large new building adjacent to their Mount Clinton Pike property and relocated their gift shop, Artisans' Hope, in bright new quarters. Artisans' Hope sells only "Fair Trade" merchandise. Fair Trade provides underemployed and unemployed artisans an opportunity to earn vital income by establishing a sustainable market for their handcrafted products.

Artisans' Hope buys approximately fifty percent of its merchandise from Ten Thousand Villages, a partner enterprise with MCC. Ten Thousand Villages has spent over sixty years cultivating long-term buying relationships in which artisans receive a fair price for their work and consumers have access to unique gifts, accessories, and home decor from around the world. In August 2009, Jay and I both began volunteering at Artisans' Hope each

Friday morning. We assist customers, arrange displays, refill the coffee bins and shelves, unpack shipments, and even water the plants in the store!

In additions to our regular work with the gift and thrift shop operations, we have helped MCC in other small ways during these retirement years. We attend comforter knotting blitzes at our church to aid in disaster relief, and one Christmas, I sewed a comforter top for our whole family to knot together on Christmas Day. Each fall, I either bake pecan pies here at home or go to the church kitchen to help Elsie with her sixty rhubarb pies for the MCC Relief Sale. We help to serve the plate lunch there on Saturday, and we eat and buy things at the auction all "for a good cause," of course! We have packed many school kits, disaster relief kits, and AIDS kits for MCC both as a family and as a church project. Each time we do another small scale "down-sizing" in our home or closets, we haul the carload of donations to an MCC thrift store drop-off location. We make donations to MCC directly and through our church budget.

All of this together is still inconsequential in light of the enormity of the world's needs. As I dust a shelf of onyx items from Pakistan, I need to keep the big picture in perspective. Only when our small bits are collected with the small bits of many others can we together help MCC make a difference.

I return to the parable of Jesus and the warning against selfishly "eating, drinking, and being merry." At the same time, I am reminded of Saint Paul's letter to the church at Corinth. "So whether you eat or drink or whatever you do, do it for the glory of God." (I Corinthians 10:31 NIV)

Can I drink for the glory of God? Yes, by buying Fair Trade coffee! Appreciating the extra time retirement offers, we have the leisure to enjoy our morning cup of some fragrant roast from Ethiopia, Peru, Columbia, or other coffee growing lands. At the same time, we sip the satisfaction of knowing that our two cups each morning increase the annual income of some small farmer and help to put in place tools for his self-sufficiency. Small farmers use organic methods which are better for our health and friendly to our environment.

Can I eat for the glory of God? Yes, again! In 1976, the *More-with-Less Cookbook* by Doris Janzen Longacre was commissioned by MCC in response to world food needs. In her introduction, Longacre writes, "There is a way, I discovered, of wasting less, eating less, and spending less which gives not less, but more." (p. 12) This way is by eating less calories, less protein, less fats, less sugar, and less super-processed foods. In this way, we use less of the world's limited resources.

The book offers easy-to-make wholesome recipes gathered from the United States and around the world. I have been influenced by the book's principles and have used many recipes since it was first printed in 1976. In retirement, I enjoy more time to "cook from scratch" and more time to savor the difference!

After Longacre publicized the plan for this cookbook, she received thousands of recipes from all over the world for consideration and testing. In the "Vegetables" chapter, she writes that she received "more recipes for zucchini than any other vegetable." (p. 219) One of these, "Zucchini Egg Foo Yung" inspired the Chinese omelet given here.

ZUCCHINI EGG FOO YUNG

Brown Sauce

Combine in saucepan:

1 cup of chicken broth
2 tablespoons lite soy sauce
1 tablespoon cornstarch

Cook and stir over low heat until thickened. Keep warm while cooking the omelet.

Omelet

Mix together in a bowl:

3 eggs, lightly beaten
¼ cup flour
¼ teaspoon garlic powder
½ teaspoon salt
2 to 3 tablespoons grated onion

Add and mix lightly:

2 medium unpeeled zucchini, grated coarsely
1 cup canned* bean sprouts, well-rinsed

*fresh bean sprouts can harbor bacteria that may cause food poisoning

Drop by large tablespoons into hot oiled skillet (or one large pancake), turning once when golden brown.

Arrange on platter and top with brown sauce.

Serve with rice. Serves four.

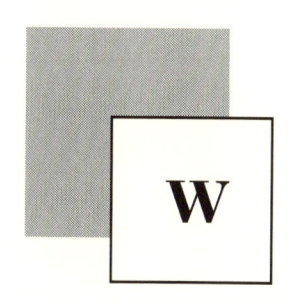

W \'də-bəl-(,)yü, də-bə-; 'dəb-(,)yü, -yə; 'dəb-yē\
n. (pl. ws or w's)
the twenty-third letter of the alphabet

WORK WRAP-UP

Recipe: Chicken Tostadas

WORK WRAP-UP

The iconic painting by Grant Wood, *American Gothic,* is sometimes viewed as an image of the Protestant work ethic. The man's pitchfork suggests hard labor, and the woman's apron and the flowers over her shoulder signify domesticity. Some see the painting as a satire poking fun at rural small-town life, while others believe it to be a depiction of the Puritan ethic and its virtues. Wood's response to some backlash regarding his work was, "All the good ideas I've ever had came to me while I was milking a cow."

I was raised on a farm—although I never really milked a cow—and the values of hard work were daily modeled by my parents along with the accompanying virtues of honesty, reliability, initiative, and accountability. When I was found reading a book instead of cleaning my bedroom, as I had been assigned, I was reminded to "get busy." To this day, I find it hard to read for pleasure during the daylight hours!

"What I want to be when I grow up" evolved from a third-grade experience in which my much admired teacher, Mrs. Mundy, left me to read stories to my classmates one afternoon when she needed to be absent from the room for a while. I liked school, and I warmed to her confidence in me. I wanted to be a teacher like Mrs. Mundy.

My dream persisted, although it shifted to the secondary level when I realized that my favorite subjects were languages and literature. In the last semester before my college graduation, I received a letter (still in my file!) from Wilbur S. Pence, superintendent of Rockingham County Public Schools. "We will probably need a Latin and English teacher for Turner Ashby High School for the session 1961 to 1962," he wrote.

None of the college education classes really prepare a beginning teacher for how much hard work goes into that first year of teaching; if the books dared to do that, there would undoubtedly be fewer teachers! Every day, I showed up in the long second-story classroom flanked on my left by a room-length bulletin board that constantly begged for redecoration and on my right by a wall of windows offering scenic distractions if my lesson became dull. I wore skirts and high heels every day and stood at the lectern facing five rows of young high school students facing me. I was "Mrs. Landis," and even the teachers addressed each other with proper titles and surnames in those days. I learned the Latin I thought I already knew. I survived the challenges of Ritchie, the brilliant class clown, and Terry, the sullen low-achiever who hated English class. I loved my Latin students, mostly bright teens who *elected* to take Latin and understood the merits of a classical language.

I became pregnant the second semester of my second year and sent back unsigned the continuing contract I was offered. My due date was the coming November. However, Latin teachers were hard to find. When Principal Yowell asked me to continue teaching part-time with only two sections of Latin, I had a decision to make.

In 1960, only one in five women with children under six held paid jobs. Prior to that time, most of the American society believed that a woman could either have a career or stay home and have children—there was no way she could do both. However, deep cultural changes were altering the role of women. In 1960, the Food and Drug Administration approved the birth control pill. In 1961, President Kennedy created the President's Commission on the Status of Women, chaired by Eleanor Roosevelt. In 1963, Betty Friedan published *The Feminine Mystique,* and in 1964, the Civil Rights Act prohibited discrimination in the workplace based on gender.

I was certainly affected by the women's movement but oblivious at the same time. I just knew that I liked to teach and that we needed the money, so I signed the contract for a half-time position and began the school year in September 1963 looking very pregnant.

When twins were born in November, I stayed on maternity leave until January. For the next year and a half, Aunt Ruby and two-year-old cousin Keith came to our house every morning to care for Ann and Jill. After Kim was born, a young woman named Marlene cared for the girls, also at our house. For six years, I taught Latin in the morning and graded papers or planned at my own dining room table in the afternoon while Jill and Ann napped or played. I felt a little guilt if they cried as I left, yet I knew they were in good care. Occasionally, I felt some condemnation from others; I remember one discussion at church in which two women spoke pointedly against "working mothers" with glances in my direction.

When Ann and Jill were ready for first grade, I had another decision to make. It seemed we were always stretching our combined salaries to barely cover our expenses. Jay applied for a position at Harrisonburg High School where the salaries were higher and was offered a job, but I knew his heart was at Eastern Mennonite College, so I applied to teach full-time at John W. Wayland Intermediate School where I taught English to eighth graders for the next four years.

Those ten years (6 PT Latin and 4 at JWW) were the best of my fifteen-year teaching career. During those years, I also worked on my master's degree and was able to apply new ideas directly in my classroom. One year when a student-teacher was assigned to me, I had time to create an individualized poetry unit that charmed even some of the most unlikely eighth-grade boys into believing they liked poetry and could write it!

During 1968 to 1969 and again from 1974 to 1976, our family lived in Idaho (see earlier chapters). Two of those three years I worked in paraprofessional roles. In 1968 to 1969, I was employed as a kindergarten teacher in a day care center for the children of Mexican-American farm laborers. In 1974 to 1975, I taught a corrective reading class and assisted in the office and library of the elementary school which Jill and Ann attended. Those were good years.

My last year of teaching in a city junior high school was my worst. I was paid more than three times my starting salary, but it wasn't enough. Hired just one week before classes began, I felt I was always scrambling to keep ahead. Conflict existed on several levels in the school. Good discipline was sometimes a challenge. I was homesick for Virginia. I hated getting up in the morning. I promised myself that I didn't have to do this the rest of my life, and even though it shook my identity, I decided to leave teaching at the end of that year.

My next career phase introduced me to *The Three Boxes of Life*, a book written by Richard Nelson Bolles (Ten Speed Press, 1981). Bolles named the three boxes "Education," "Work," and "Retirement" and proposed that they correspond roughly to a person's life span. From birth to age eighteen or twenty-two, a person focuses on education with some play but very little work. For the next forty to forty-five years, the emphasis is on work with some job-related education and just enough play to avoid complete burnout. In the retirement stage, the overemphasis is on leisure with little formal education or employment.

My Box of Work extended from age twenty-two when I graduated from college to age sixty-two when I took an early retirement, a period of forty years. Within my Work Box are three distinct compartments. The first compartment of fifteen years was labeled "Teaching." When I decided to leave teaching, I discovered that the lid on the box was not tight, that one could escape to a new career, maybe even more than once in a lifetime.

The second compartment in my Work Box is labeled "Student Life," and its contents span a seventeen-year period of employment in higher education at Eastern Mennonite College. They hired me as director of career development for what they believed I could do, not for what I already knew or had done in the past. My role as a career advisor was to help young adults step out of their education boxes and into work boxes.

I learned that I myself had "transferable skills," abilities I brought with me from my teaching which could be put to use in a new situation. I used my ability to instruct others in workshop presentations about job search skills, and I taught how to draft a résumé and prepare for an interview. My ability to plan helped me organize job fairs and set up interview schedules with employers. I used my ability to solve problems as I advised undeclared majors about a program of study that they would both enjoy and find marketable. My skills in written communications helped me produce a newsletter for seniors called *Keys* which gave information about available positions, and my ability to locate and classify information directed me in the development of a small career library of books and other materials. One semester, I taught secondary methods in education for a professor on sabbatical leave, and I directed the Continuing Education program for community adults for several years. I was also named director of testing and administered professional batteries such as the MCAT (Medical College Admissions Test).

"Follow your bliss, and the universe will open doors where there were only walls," Joseph Campbell once recommended and career counselors have often echoed. I was happy in my work in higher education during those eight years and was exploring the possibility of earning a doctor's degree when I was invited to make a shift within the Student Life Division.

The college was awarded a federal Title III grant for an integrated students services project and the director of our student life division wanted to step aside and administer the grant while he completed his doctoral dissertation. I agreed to take the director of student life position which began on an interim basis and eventually grew into a permanent role.

This was definitely a step up, and I took it with some trepidation. In my Work Box, I find some journaling I did on my first day in October 1983. "The past month has called for much reflection and introspection. I think all the signals were "go," although I must admit that the color green was dim and flickered at times ... God bless people like Marie Shenk. I had just walked into my new office and was feeling like an intruder. She said, "Welcome to Northlawn. I'm glad you're here." Her tone was warm and genuine, and it made the tremors ease a little ... Erma was kind and helpful. We need to establish our working relationship. That has probably been my number one anxiety—woman working with woman where one has risen above her peer and the salary reflects it, yet the assistant knows more about the job ... "

On the second day, the job began to take shape, and I wrote, "I talked with Miriam and Don about insurance concerns, with Carey about an off-campus housing problem, with Joe about a sick student. I attended my first President's Cabinet meeting. I've always imagined that high level, institution-shaping discussions are taking place behind those closed doors, but I actually felt kind of sleepy several times ... A student is dropping out. God wants her to, she says, so that she can 'grow in Him!' How can I be supportive of her faith yet help her recognize that her problem is homesickness? Two students up and got married last weekend, a freshman boy had a malignant testicle removed, an attorney's office called, looking to get in touch with a student ... "

"The end of the first week! I'm surprised that I feel as calm about it all as I do. My biggest concern—Erma—has largely diminished. She is a good sport and has certainly been a great help to me. One day, she told me that she is determined to show people that two women *can* work together ... Representing student life on important committees seems to be a large portion of my job. The planning action team has been in session deciding how to cover a two-hundred-thousand-dollar-gap in the budget projections . . . Tonight was open house in the dorms. I helped judge the "Express Yourself" contest in five dorms. It was a good chance to see the Halls, but—oh—my feet!"

The days and years moved on, never two alike. Sometimes I just wished for a boring day! My responsibilities included recruiting, supervising, and evaluating a fourteen-member staff who headed the offices of housing, residence life, campus ministries, multicultural programs, career development, counseling, health, and student activities. I developed long-range plans, monitored budgets, reported regularly to constituent groups, and was a member of the President's Cabinet. I developed a first-year experience course for all freshmen. When it came to tough discipline decisions, the ball was in my court.

The year 1990 to 1991 was an *annus horribilis* when death and tragedy traumatized the campus too many times. Student unrest caused by the beginning of the Gulf War was followed by the murder of a student's parents, an alleged rape, the unexpected death of a student because of a heart defect, and the suicide of one from our division.

My edges were becoming frayed. The following December, Erma, who had become a close friend and my wonderful coworker/assistant, resigned to join George in his sabbatical work. Jay and I were scheduled to lead our second semester-long cross-cultural trip to Great Britain in the fall of 1992. I resigned in June 1992 without a plan for myself beyond the semester in England.

The following kind action by the Board of Trustees felt like a balm and a blessing.

Action XIII. For eight years Peggy H. Landis has brought

- communication skills,
- creativity,
- graciousness,
- wisdom,
- sense of humor,
- enabling skills

to her role as director of Student Life.

These gifts, coupled with her faith and administration skills, mark her tenure as "exceptional."

We wish her well as she discerns God's leading for the next stages of her life. (Hess/Mumaw)

When we returned from Great Britain, Jay had a second semester sabbatical, and I decided to take one too. It was time to retool before I opened the third compartment in my Work Box. We bought our first home computer, and I enrolled in a three-hour credit course at Blue Ridge Community College to learn word processing. Until then, I had sat at my desk and written everything in long hand and given it to a secretary to keyboard for me. Those were the days before all executives and managers carried laptops in their briefcases.

Later that spring, the telephone rang, and I heard an unfamiliar voice from Goshen, Indiana. Dean Preheim-Bartel from Mennonite Mutual Aid (now Everence) had learned that I might be available, and the company had a need for a fraternal advisor. I was familiar with MMA, the insurance and financial services agency of the Mennonite Church. We had health insurance with them, and they also managed the Mennonite Retirement Trust in which our pension funds were lodged. But what was a "fraternal advisor"?

I learned that MMA's unique tax status as a "fraternal benefits organization" allowed the company to distribute monies, that would have otherwise been paid in taxes, to persons in need through member congregations. The Sharing Fund, a matching grant program, relied on a system of "advocates" in each congregation who were serviced by a resource and communications link called a fraternal advisor (now called a church relations representative). Fraternal advisors were assigned to regional areas, and my area covered Virginia, West Virginia, North Carolina, Maryland, and Washington DC. There were nine fraternal advisors located throughout the United States.

Thus, the third compartment in my Work Box was labeled "Church Relations/Public Relations." The business environment was distinctly different than my previous work in the education sector had been and required a lot more data keeping. The computer course I had just taken was swiftly put to use. My colleagues in the local office were a regional sales manager, a Mennonite Foundation representative, several MMA counselors (sales agents), and an office assistant. There were regular telephone appointments with my supervisor in Indiana and frequent teleconferences that linked home office personnel with fraternal advisors, always at a time convenient for both east and west coast offices.

Travel became an important aspect of the work, and I kept a suitcase partially packed for my quarterly trips to the home office in Indiana and occasional overnights to meet with pastors and advocates in my more distant areas. The fraternal advisors were invited to the company's annual sales conferences, and we enjoyed weekends in cities such as Columbus, Indianapolis, Kansas City, Pittsburgh, and South Bend.

My work with nearly one hundred churches introduced me to compassionate advocates who volunteered for the sheer joy of helping someone with unexpected medical bills or living expenses during a time of need. Caring pastors welcomed this assistance for their members as well as our resources for stewardship education and healthy living. In a typical year, MMA might award grants to more than two thousand families nationwide, the total, coupled with the matching funds, exceeding several million dollars. It was so much fun to give away money!

MMA was a good employer, and many times, I was on the receiving end. In addition to the satisfaction of working with great colleagues for such a significant cause, I was also rewarded in other ways. At precisely the right time in my life, I learned more about retirement planning, including 401(k) savings, mutual fund investing, and long-term care insurance.

After eight years with MMA (Everence), I decided it was time to move outside of the Work Box, that was never too confining for a person who enjoys working, to a period of self-employment otherwise known as retirement. I needed to give more time to my mother who was not well, enjoy my grandchildren, and explore some personal interests.

Author Richard Nelson Bolles wrote *The Three Boxes of Life* to encourage his readers to balance education, employment, and recreation throughout the life span. My Work Box was not equally balanced, but it did include learning and leisure which often lightened the work load.

Always, my coworkers were ready to celebrate milestones and achievements, none more so than the jovial Student Life staff. One year when school had finally ended, we celebrated our survival on Helen's new deck in Belmont. The meal was another team effort—a tostada buffet with contributions from everyone's kitchen. Val remembered how her mother fried the tortillas, and she brought the crispy shells. Gerald's dishpan full of shredded lettuce could have served the whole student body! I remember making the Mexican coffee with chocolate, cinnamon, and whipped cream. Who brought each of the other items is long lost, but the solidarity of the occasion is not forgotten.

CHICKEN TOSTADAS

Tostada Shells
8 corn tortillas
Cooking spray

Preheat oven to 375 degrees. Spray tortillas on both sides with cooking spray. Place on baking sheet and into oven. Bake for eight to ten minutes or until crispy, turning once.

Refried Beans

3 tablespoons butter
2 cans (15 and ½ oz.) red kidney beans with liquid
¼ cup onion, chopped fine
1 clove garlic, minced
2 tablespoons chopped green chilies
½ teaspoon ground cumin
salt to taste

Melt butter in large frying pan; sauté onion, garlic, and pepper until tender. Add beans with liquid and mash with a fork. Add salt and cumin. Simmer ten to fifteen minutes on low heat to blend flavors.

Tostada Chicken Filling

2 tablespoons margarine or butter
¼ cup onion, chopped fine
3 cups chicken breast, skinned, cooked, shredded with two forks
16 oz. can tomato sauce
1 teaspoon sugar
½ teaspoon salt
1 teaspoon chili powder
¼ teaspoon cumin

In large skillet, melt margarine; sauté onion until tender. Add chicken and remaining ingredients. Simmer for twenty to thirty minutes, stirring occasionally, until flavors are well blended.

Choice of Toppings

Romaine lettuce shredded
Tomatoes, chopped
Monterey Jack and cheddar cheeses, shredded
Ripe olives, sliced

Low sodium salsa
Fresh cilantro, chopped
Sliced avocado or guacamole
Fresh lime wedges

To Serve

Place toppings in separate bowls. Bring out tostada shells from the oven in batches, keeping unused ones warm in the oven. Invite guests to serve themselves from buffet table. To prepare the tostada, each person should spread a large spoonful of mashed beans over the tostada shell first, then add chicken and cheese and whatever toppings desired. Best not to overload the tostada too much, or it will be difficult to eat.

Eat by picking up the tostada with two hands (like a pizza slice). This is definitely a two-napkin meal!

Serves six to eight.

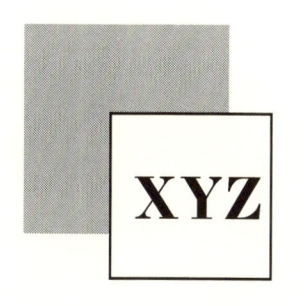

XYZ \'eks\, \'wī\, \'zē\ (also x, y, z) n. (pl. xs or x's, ys or y's, zs or z's) the last three letters of the alphabet

XYZ: A CONCLUSION

Recipe: Chocolate Swirl Cheesecake

XYZ: A CONCLUSION

The bell rang for class to begin, and our prim, diminutive teacher stood with her back half visible to the eighth grade algebra class, reached as high as she could to write the equation on the blackboard and said, "Let x stand for the unknown."

Years before her, Descartes, seventeenth century French philosopher and mathematician, stood before his analytic geometry class and declared that the first three letters of the alphabet should stand for known quantities, and the last three, X, Y, Z, should stand for unknown quantities. To this point, I have detailed the "known" quantities—the ABCs of my life. From here, as the hymn writer penned, "the future all unknown . . . ," the XYZs are a blank page.

In 1998, Jay and I took a short summer vacation in the state of Kentucky. Our most memorable stop was at the monastic community of the Abbey of Gethsemani at Trappist, Kentucky. Here, Thomas Merton, known as Father Louis in the monastery, spent the years 1941 to 1968 writing about the contemplative life, prayer, social problems and Christian responsibility, and the lives of spiritual leaders. His own autobiography, *The Seven Storey Mountain*, was first published in 1948 by Harcourt Brace and Company.

We attended Sext, the noontime service of the Liturgy of the Hours, sitting in a high balcony at the back of the long nave, a place reserved for visitors. The monks in flowing white robes entered in solemn procession to read from the psalms, sing, and pray.

On a sloping hillside outside the church and overlooking the valley and woodlands below, we stood by the small white metal cross, exactly the same as all the others with a grave marker that read "Father Louis Merton, died December 10, 1968."

In the gift shop, we browsed the racks of literature, enjoyed the carved sculptures and paintings, and were tempted by the cheese, fruitcake, and bourbon fudge which the monks make and sell to supplement their income from the farm. I bought a simple card with a quotation from Merton's *Thoughts in Solitude*.

> *My Lord God,* I have no idea where I am going. I do not see the road ahead of me. I cannot know for certain where it will end. Nor do I really know myself, and the fact that I think that I am following your will does not mean that I am actually doing so. But I believe that the desire to please you does in fact please you. And I hope I have that desire in all that I am doing. I hope that I will never do anything apart from that desire. And I know that if I do this, you will lead me by the right road, although I may know nothing about

it. Therefore, I will trust you always, although I may seem to be lost and in the shadow of death. I will not fear, for you are ever with me, and you will never leave me to face my perils alone.

This timeless prayer, known as "The Merton Prayer," has been translated into many languages and prayed throughout the world. It gives comfort and assurance to each believer who faces the XYZs of his and her existence. I, like Thomas Merton who died accidentally by electrocution in Thailand "do not see the road ahead of me," but "will not fear, for you are ever with me . . ."

"Life is short—eat dessert first!" is a quotation variously attributed to Katherine Hepburn, Ogden Nash, Mark Twain, and Sue Ellen Cooper, founder of the Red Hat Society. It has *not* been my guiding principle.

A few years ago, I threw away a jar of lemon curd that had been pushed to the back of a cupboard shelf. A friend had once given it to me for Christmas, pale yellow cream glowing through the pretty octagonal glass jar. I saved it, I believe, for some future special occasion, but while I waited for that perfect time, the lemon curd separated and became discolored.

While I do not advocate eating dessert first, I do believe that one should eat dessert and eat it rather often. My advice to myself and others regarding future gifts of "lemon curd" is to enjoy it! The present time *is* a special time and worthy of celebration!

Chocolate swirl cheesecake is a special dessert. Make it soon! Invite family or friends and celebrate, whatever the season.

CHOCOLATE SWIRL CHEESECAKE

Crust

1 and ¾ cups chocolate wafer crumbs
¼ cup sugar
⅓ cup butter, melted

In a small bowl, combine cookie crumbs and sugar; stir in butter. Reserve one fourth cup of the crumbs for topping. Press the remaining crumbs into the bottom and one and a half inches up the sides of a greased nine-inch springform pan. Place pan on a baking sheet. Bake at 350 degrees for ten minutes. Place pan on a wire rack to cool.

Filling

3 eight-ounce packages cream cheese, softened
1 cup sugar
1 tablespoon vanilla
4 eggs
2 teaspoons grated orange peel
2 one-ounce squares semisweet chocolate, melted and cooled

Beat together cream cheese and sugar. Add vanilla, eggs, and orange peel. Beat well until smooth.

Set aside three-fourth cup; pour remaining filling into the pan. Combine melted chocolate and reserved filling. Drop small amounts onto the cake batter in a random pattern. Cut through the batter several times (not too often) with a knife to swirl in the filling.

Sprinkle with reserved crumbs. Bake on baking sheet in 350-degree oven for about forty minutes or until center is almost set. Cool pan on a wire rack for ten minutes. Carefully run a knife around edge of pan to loosen; cool one hour longer. Refrigerate overnight.

Serving

chocolate syrup
fresh red raspberries
whipped cream

Stripe serving plates with chocolate syrup. Remove sides of springform pan and slice cheesecake. Place slice on the chocolate stripping and top with raspberries and whipped cream. Makes twelve to sixteen servings.

Recipe Index

Soups and Salads
Arlene's Potato Soup, 33
Dandelion Salad with Hot Bacon Dressing, 68
Lentil Soup, 143
Mandarin Strawberry Salad, 95
My Chicken Corn Soup, 161
Split Pea Soup with Barley, 41
Swiss Cashew Tossed Salad, 95
Turkey and Squash Soup, 119

Breads and Grains
Blueberry Oatmeal Muffins, 182
Blueberry-Stuffed French Toast, 94
Cherry Cream Scones, 61
My Granola, 188
Orange-Date Pumpkin Muffins, 146
Pumpkin Bread, 86
Sourdough Starter, 133
Sourdough Bread or Rolls, 134
Sourdough Pancakes, 135

Meats and Main Dishes
Baked Burritos, 128
Baked Salmon Filets Dijon, 94
Chicken and Asparagus Frittata, 51
Chicken Tostadas, 275
Curried Chicken Divan, 203
Ham Potpie, 19
Moussaka, 81

Oven-Fried Chicken, 111
Oyster Dressing, 39
Skillet-Fried Chicken, 110
Sugar-Cured Country Ham, 102
Turkey Curry, 120

Vegetable and Side Dishes
Corn Pudding (Jill), 248
Five-Cheese, Five-Vegetable Lasagna, 211
Fried Apples, 51
Ratatouille, 69
Rebecca's Sweet Potato Cranberry Bake, 228
Savory Squash Bake (Ann), 248
Zucchini Egg Foo Yung, 264

Desserts
Chocolate Swirl Cheesecake, 282
Fresh Fruit with Orange Glaze, 17
Peach and Berry Crisp, 176
Pink Baked Apples, 169
Soft Egg Custard, 47

Cakes, Cookies, and Pastries
Applesauce Cake, 25
Aunt Alice's Old-Fashioned Sugar Cookies, 257
McIntosh Oatmeal Cookies, 153
Medium Dark Fruitcake, 36

Raspberry Cream Cheese Cake, 27
Strawberry Shortcake, 233
Thimbleberry Pie, 240

Specials
A "Proper" Pot of Tea, 61
Ann's Fruit Smoothie, 85
Cracker Jack, 141
Orange-Blueberry Freezer Jam, 183
Poppy Seed Salad Dressing, 95
Rose Petals (candied), 218
Rose Petal Potpourri (nonedible), 219
Rose Petal Tea, 218

Made in the USA
Lexington, KY
13 April 2013